BERICHTE AUS DEM PRODUKTIONSTECHNISCHEN ZENTRUM BERLIN

Jochen Radmer

Depth Data based Determination of Gait Parameters of Subjects after Stroke for the Use in Clinical Gait Rehabilitation

Fraunhofer IPK
INSTITUT PRODUKTIONSANLAGEN UND KONSTRUKTIONSTECHNIK

IWF
INSTITUT WERKZEUGMASCHINEN UND FABRIKBETRIEB
TECHNISCHE UNIVERSITÄT BERLIN

Kontaktadresse:
Fraunhofer-Institut für Produktionsanlagen und Konstruktionstechnik IPK
Pascalstraße 8-9
10587 Berlin
Telefon 030 39006-0
Fax 030 39110-37
E-Mail info@ipk.fraunhofer.de
URL www.ipk.fraunhofer.de

Bibliografische Information der Deutschen Nationalbibliothek
Die Deutsche Nationalbibliothek verzeichnet diese Publikation in der Deutschen Nationalbibliografie; detaillierte bibliografische Daten sind im Internet über http://dnb.d-nb.de abrufbar.
ISBN: 978-3-8396-0332-1

D 83

Zugl.: Berlin, TU, Diss., 2011

Druck: Mediendienstleistungen des
Fraunhofer-Informationszentrum Raum und Bau IRB, Stuttgart

Für den Druck des Buches wurde chlor- und säurefreies Papier verwendet.

Fraunhofer-Informationszentrum Raum und Bau IRB
Postfach 800469, 70504 Stuttgart
Nobelstraße 12, 70569 Stuttgart
Telefon 0711 970-2500
Fax 0711 970-2508
E-Mail verlag@fraunhofer.de
URL http://verlag.fraunhofer.de

Depth Data based Determination of Gait Parameters of Subjects after Stroke for the Use in Clinical Gait Rehabilitation

von Diplom-Ingenieur
Jochen Radmer
aus Berlin

von der Fakultät V – Verkehrs- und Maschinensysteme
der Technischen Universität Berlin
zur Erlangung des akademischen Grades

Doktor der Ingenieurwissenschaften
– Dr.-Ing. –

genehmigte Dissertation

Promotionsausschuss:
Vorsitzender: Prof. Dr.-Ing. Rainer Stark
Gutachter: Prof. Dr.-Ing. Jörg Krüger
Gutachter: Prof. Dr.-Ing. Alexander Verl

Tag der wissenschaftlichen Aussprache: 8. Juni 2011

Berlin 2011
D 83

Depth Data based Determination of Gait Parameters of Subjects after Stroke for the Use in Clinical Gait Rehabilitation

vorgelegt von
Dipl.-Ing. Jochen Radmer

von
der Fakultät V - Verkehrs- und Maschinensysteme
der Technischen Universität Berlin
zur Erlangung des akademischen Grades

Doktor der Ingenieurwissenschaften
- Dr.-Ing. -

genehmigte Dissertation

Promotionsausschuss:

Chairman:	Prof. Dr.-Ing. Rainer Stark
Reviewer:	Prof. Dr.-Ing. Jörg Krüger
Reviewer:	Prof. Dr.-Ing. Alexander Verl

Day of the scientific debate 08.06.2011

Berlin,
D83

Danksagung

Ich danke Prof. Dr.-Ing. Jörg Krüger für seine Unterstützung, sein Vertrauen und die wissenschaftlichen Freiheiten, die er mir während meiner Zeit an seinem Lehrstuhl gewährte. Mein Dank gilt zudem Prof. Dr.-Ing. Alexander Verl für die Übernahme des Koreferats sowie Prof. Dr.-Ing. Rainer Stark für den Vorsitz.

Danken möchte ich außerdem allen meinen Kollegen und Studenten, insbesondere jedoch Sami Hussein und Udo Templiner als Kollegen der ersten Stunde, durch die ich nicht zuletzt meine Musikkenntnisse zu den Spielarten des Metal entscheidend erweitern konnte und nun auch *'fantasy power metal'* einzuordnen verstehe.

Markus Schwarz und Frank Partey als gute Freunde und meine gesamte Familie unterstützten mich durch das Korrekturlesen dieser Arbeit. Herauszuheben sind dabei meine Schwester Christine Deeken und mein Bruder Stephan Radmer, der mit einer unglaublichen Gründlichkeit jeden Satz dieser Arbeit in Frage stellte. Katja Eschke danke ich darüber hinaus für die hingebungsvolle Unterstützung und die schönen Jahre während dieser Arbeit.

Abstract

Stroke often results in long term care. The personal consequences of the individual as well as the economical consequences for the society are enormous. Because of the demographic development, the amount of stroke patients of now approx. 250 000 incidents only in Germany will further increase. This leads to an immense future burden on the health systems. Health insurances increasingly need to apply a 'cost vs. benefit' analysis for medical interventions. Therefore, the benefit of a treatment continuously needs to be measured and documented.

After the acute treatment stroke patients often need a long lasting rehabilitation treatment. The aim must therefore be to make the therapy as effective as possible in order to put the patient in the position to participate in active life. Important for this is to regain unassisted mobility.

An approach to achieve this is the continuous patient-adaptive gait therapy, in which the therapy progress is measured and provided to the therapists to adjust the therapy accordingly. Currently available systems have disadvantages. Therefore, systems must be developed which reliably measure the gait quality and meet the requirements to be widely applicable in clinical environment.

In this work a system is presented that provides a measure for the gait quality through joint angle trajectories and that aims to meet the requirements for wide clinical applicability. As sensory basis a Time of Flight (TOF) camera is chosen. This sensor has not yet been applied by any other research group for the determination of gait parameters. Because the depth data provided by the TOF camera out-of-the-box is not applicable for gait parameter determination, novel calibration methods have been developed to enhance the depth data so that they meet the requirements of the considered task. The method applies a model-based approach to capture the body movement from a sequence of depth images. A body model is parameterized so that it corresponds to the depth data and therefore reflects the body posture of the patient. The joint angle trajectories are derived from the course of the body model posture over the time. To cover also rotational movements that are not represented by the depth data, corners are identified in 3D and tracked across several images.

Kurzfassung

Schlaganfälle führen oft zu einer dauerhaften Pflegebedürftigkeit. Sowohl die sozialen Folgen des Einzelnen als auch die ökonomischen Folgen für die Gesellschaft sind enorm. Aufgrund der demographischen Entwicklung wird die Anzahl der Schlaganfallpatienten von gegenwärtig allein in Deutschland jährlich rund 250.000 Fällen weiter steigen. Damit verbunden ist eine immense zukünftige Belastung der Gesundheitssysteme. Dies führt dazu, dass zunehmend eine Kosten/Nutzenanalyse für medizinische Maßnahmen zugrunde gelegt wird. Ein Ansatzpunkt hierzu ist die evidenzbasierte Medizin, die eine nachgewiesene Wirksamkeit für jede medizinische Behandlung verlangt. Diese Arbeit versucht hierzu einen Beitrag zu leisten.

Schlaganfallpatienten benötigen nach einer ersten akuten Versorgung häufig eine langwierige Rehabilitationsmaßnahme. Im Vordergrund steht hierbei, die eigenständige Mobilität so weit wie möglich wieder herzustellen.
Ein Ansatz, dies zu erreichen, ist die kontinuierliche patientenadaptive Gangtherapie, bei der laufend der Therapiefortschritt jedes Patienten erfasst und dem Therapeuten zur Anpassung der Therapie bereitgestellt wird. Die hierfür momentan zur Verfügung stehenden Systeme weisen jedoch Nachteile auf. Daher müssen Systeme entwickelt werden, die die Gangqualität zuverlässig erfassen und den Anforderungen für einen breiten Einsatz im klinischen Umfeld entsprechen.

In dieser Arbeit wird ein System vorgestellt, dass die Gangqualität über Gelenkwinkelverläufe als Gangparameter erfasst und das unter Berücksichtigung der Anforderungen für einen breiten Einsatz im klinischen Umfeld. Als sensorielle Basis wird hierzu erstmals eine Tiefenkamera gewählt. Dieser Sensor wurde bisher von keiner anderen Forschungsgruppe für die Bestimmung von Gelenkwinkelverläufen verwendet. Da die Tiefendaten nicht die Genauigkeitsanforderungen für die Gangparameterbestimmung erfüllen, werden neuartige Kalibrierverfahren entwickelt, um dies zu erreichen. Das Verfahren verwendet einen modellbasierten Ansatz zur Erfassung der Körperbewegung aus aufeinander folgenden Tiefenbildern. Dazu wird ein räumliches Körpermodell so parametriert, dass es den Tiefendaten und somit der Körperhaltung des Patienten entspricht. Die Gelenkwinkelverläufe werden aus der zeitlichen Abfolge der Modellkörperhaltung abgeleitet. Um auch rotatorische Bewegungen zu erfassen, die sich nicht in Tiefendaten abbilden, werden Merkmale im 3D identifiziert und über mehrere Aufnahmen hinweg verfolgt.

Contents

1 Introduction

1.1 Motivation - Present Situation - Gait Analysis of Stroke Patients in the Clinical Gait Rehabilitation

Damages of the human central nervous system (CNS) form the main cause for mobility restrictions and motor impediment [50]. These damages are caused by stroke with in Germany about 250 000 impairments per year. As a result of the stroke the majority of the patients must cope with paralysis up to an entire loss of the voluntary motor control. Due to this many are not able to move themselves autonomously or to lead an independent life anymore. They need a wheel chair and permanent support for everyday life. With the demographic development the number of the stroke patients will further rise in coming decades. Serious social and economic consequences arise out of this for the situation of the social security systems.
After the acute treatment the rehabilitation is carried out for about several weeks to months. Thereby, the patient slowly relearns movements of the affected arms, hands and legs by special therapy exercises (see figure 1.1). The success of this rehabilitation treatment determines on whether the patient is afterwards able to lead a widely independent life and to achieve a re-integration. But just 80% of the patients regain a minimum in independent walking ability on even grounds at the end of the stationary rehabilitation (e. g., gait security when climbing stairs, walking on uneven ground, tripping and slipping). These patients are far from an everyday walking ability and need at least partial nursing. Therefore, a more efficient and effective gait therapy is needed.

A key to achieve this is to measure and monitor the therapy progress of each patient and adapt the therapy accordingly. The therapy progress is defined by the improvement of the gait quality throughout the therapy. The gait quality is deduced from the joint angle trajectories, their symmetry and characteristics by therapist and medical staff. Therefore, these gait parameters need to be continuously determined and monitored.
To illustrate the idea of the continuous adaptive gait therapy, it can be compared with a control loop in which the actual values are continuously determined in order to adapt the control parameters in such a way that the target set point is reached. Here, the actual gait

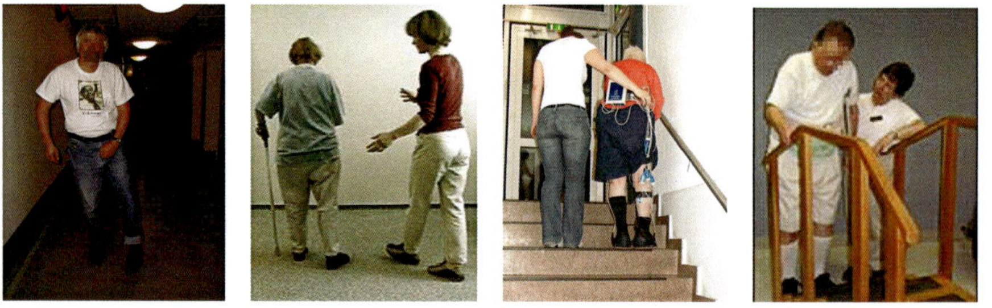

Figure 1.1: Different walking ability levels of stroke patients after stationary rehabilitation treatment (low gait security, pathologic motion patterns on even ground and stair climbing, high risk of falling) (property of Department for neurological rehabilitation, Charité Berlin).

parameters correspond to the actual values and the desired gait parameters for high gait quality correspond to the desired set point. The determination of the actual gait parameters is the crucial task of the adaptive gait therapy. Current systems that are capable to determine the gait parameters have shortcomings that inhibit their application in clinical everyday use. These drawbacks are manifold, such as time-consuming due to its set-up time, expensive or spacious. Therefore, systems for gait parameter determination need to be realized that conform to the prerequisites of a clinical everyday use. This forms the focus of this work.

To quantitatively determine the gait parameters, methods of orthopedic biomechanical gait analysis are to be used ideally. However, this is not practicable in the everyday clinical practice of rehabilitation because of the high technical and temporal expenses, as well as the demand in specially certified operating staff. Hence, almost solely qualitative scales and scores are used in medical centers by therapists for the inquiry of the therapy progress [41]. The biggest problem by the use of qualitative scales is that they are by nature subjective and show a high variance. The reason for this is a high *inter-rater variability*[1] and, additionally, a high *intra-rater variability*[2]. These both overlapping aspects result in a significant shortcoming concerning the determination of the gait parameters and the continuous diagnosis of the patient's gait deficits. In practice, it shows that the simultaneous capture and classification for the use of the scales is problematic. Due to the limited endurance of the patient there needs to be breaks to rest, which makes the visual assessment by the therapist very time consuming. Therefore, doctors and therapist wish for a system which does not show aforementioned short comings.

[1]variance in the subjectivity of the assessment by different therapists

[2]fluctuations in the assessment by the same therapist over time (e. g., at different therapy sessions)

1.2 Objective of this Work

The objective of this work is to provide a base for a gait analysis system for clinical every day use for the recognition of pathological gait patterns of stroke patients. The essential criteria of such systems are according to literature of [14] and [15]:

CRITERIA FOR CLINICAL GAIT PARAMETER DETERMINATION
• widely applicable, i. e., non-spacious and not specially equipped laboratories • short set-up time because stroke patients have limited endurance • accurate data • capable of extracting relevant gait parameters • an easy use and service by non-technical trained staff, like physiotherapists • represent gait parameters in form of accepted clinical concepts • not affecting the gait of the patients • cost-effective

The major criterion is that a system is not spacious so that it can be used in normal clinical environment. A short set-up time is another elementary feature of such a system. This is achieved by a system without the need for attaching markers to the patient's body. The omittance of markers avoids the altering of the gait. Therefore, a markerless system, which uses a Time-of-Flight (TOF) camera, is aimed to realize for gait parameter determination.

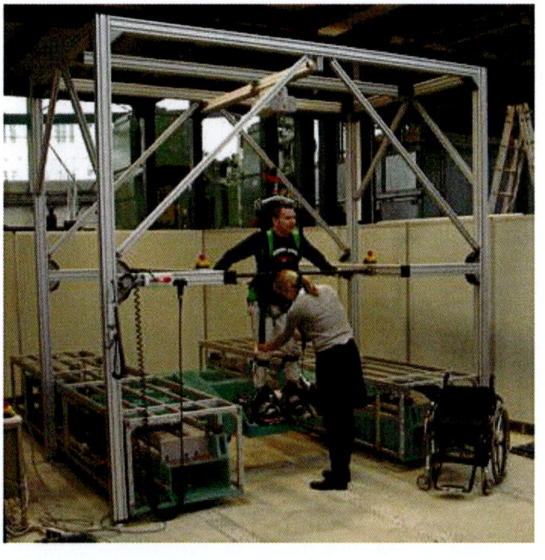

Figure 1.2: Stroke patient on the gait rehabilitation robot *HapticWalker* [92]

The measured gait parameters are the pelvis, the hip and the knee joint angles trajectories as well as the gait symmetry of the gait on the base of the pelvis' movement. These gait parameters are considered relevant for gait quality determination [23], [39], [41], [64], [76], [98]. As demonstration scenario the gait rehabilitation robot *HapticWalker*, which is shown in figure 1.2, is considered [92].

1.3 Outline

Currently the most common approach for optical gait parameter determination is the multi-camera *shape-from-silhouette* approach. This approach is very spacious and needs a unobstructed view for all cameras and, therefore, cannot cope with the bars and the weight suspension of the *HapticWalker*. A single-view approach is more advantageous. This is accounted for by choosing a Time-of-Flight (TOF) camera as sensory base because it provides depth information of a single-view without showing the systematic errors of a stereo-vision system.
Up to now no other research group implemented the TOF camera for gait parameter determination which includes the pelvic movements. Especially, the frontal view has not been incorporated for gait parameter determination so far, although the TOF camera is ideally suited for this view because it captures depth information.
Due to the novelty of the camera technology, the camera shows systematic errors that have not been fully investigated and compensated up to now. Therefore, this work also includes the enhancement of the captured depth data accuracy so that the accuracy conforms to the needs of the to-be-realized system.

This makes the TOF camera a promising sensory base for the use in clinical every day life. Furthermore, the camera forms an excellent platform for future applications, like tele-rehabilitation for home treatment.

2 State of the Art - Clinical Gait Analysis, Systems and Approaches

Within this chapter the prerequisites for the development of an optical markerless system for gait parameter determination which arise from the application in the orthopedic biomechanical analysis in clinical everyday life are worked out. Therefore, at first an overview is given including some basics and definitions about the human gait and the clinical situation starting with the human gait. Additionally, related research for gait analysis and TOF data enhancement are presented.

2.1 Biomechanical Gait Analysis

The biomechanical gait analysis consists of several disciplines. The most important are the biomechanics of sports, the ergonomic, the traumatic and the orthopedic biomechanics. The latter is considered within the scope of this work so that in the following the term *gait analysis* always corresponds to *orthopedic biomechanical gait analysis*. Gait analysis is defined in [37] as the investigation and qualitative capture of pathological structures and functions of the human movement apparatus. Additionally, it comprises methods of capturing, quantitative description, standardized diagnostics and treatment of functional disturbances in the skeletal system.

2.2 Human Gait

For the targeting development of a gait analysis system for stroke patients, it is important to know which stroke patient specific gait abnormalities appear because they define the to-be-captured movements. Therefore, within this section normal gait and gait abnormalities that are stroke patient specific are reviewed.

2.2.1 Normal Gait

For the description of human movements within the discipline of gait analysis the projection planes displayed in figure 2.1 are standardly used [75], [104], [105]. The direction and location notations are:

- *medial* (towards body center), *lateral* (away from body center);
- *anterior* (towards walking direction), *posterior* (towards back direction);
- *proximal* (close to the torso), *distal* (distant from the torso).

Additionally, the figure displays the different projection planes, *frontal* (also *coronal*), *transverse* and *sagittal*.

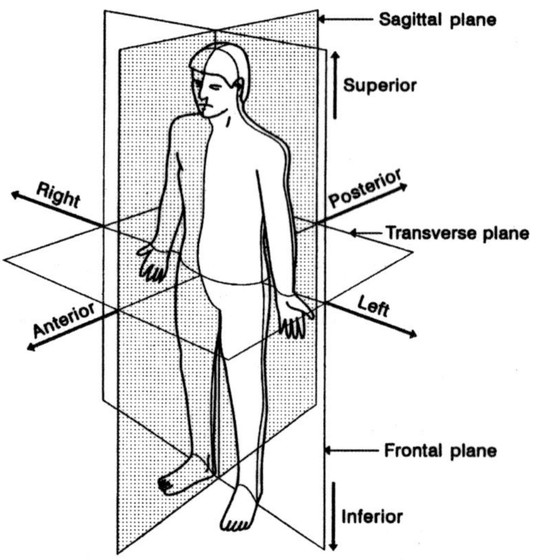

Figure 2.1: The reference projection planes of the human body in the standard anatomical position extracted from [105].

The bipedal locomotion of the human body is based on the shifting of the body center of mass (COM) through the lower extremities. The physiological gait shows a cyclic alternating movement of the body and its limbs, the gait cycle. The gait cycle comprises of several phases [75], [89], [105]. The figure 2.2 shows one gait cycle for normal floor walking.

One gait cycle, which is also called a stride, describes the motion sequence of the leg and foot of one side between two heel contacts. The stride always refers to one leg and begins with the so-called *initial heel contact* and describes two main phases, the stance phase and the swing phase phases [75], [89], [105]. In figure 2.2, the darkened right leg is taken as the referring leg, the left leg is the so-called contra lateral leg. During the stance phase the foot of the considered reference leg is in contact with the ground. In the swing phase the foot swings forward without ground contact.

On a more detailed level of abstraction one stride is divided into eight gait phases, five belonging to the stance phase and three to the swing phase. These eight phases are illustrated in figure 2.2. The relation of stance and swing phase is about 60% to 40% for walking on even ground and slightly varies for other movements like stair climbing. The stance is subdivided in [75] into two functional parts which occur subsequently. First, the *weight acceptance/double support* (0%-12%) and then the *single limb support* (12%-62%) (see figure 2.2). The *weight acceptance* starts the stance period when the body is supported by both legs. It is subdivided into the *initial heel contact* with the following weight takeover from one leg to the other which enables the subsequent *single limb support*. The *weight acceptance* period ends when the other foot starts the swing phase by leaving the ground at the *toe-off* event at 12%. During the *single limb support*, the body weight is supported by just one leg. This period is subdivided into the *middle* and *terminal stance* and part of the *pre-swing*. The period ends when the contra lateral foot contacts the floor and the second *double support* begins. After the second bilateral *double support* phase the foot starts the swing phase beginning with the *pre-swing* sequence followed by the *initial swing*, the *middle swing* and ending with the *terminal swing*. Finally, the gait cycle starts over with another *initial heel contact* [39], [76]. For the safe of completeness, it shall be mentioned that other categorizations exist.

For gait analysis the human body is divided into two functional units, namely *passenger* and *locomotor* [71]. The passenger has no direct contribution for the walking trial and consists of the upper body half: head, arms, torso and pelvis. The pelvis and the legs form the locomotor, i. e., the pelvis belongs to both as a connecting element. Nevertheless, as connecting element the pelvic movement plays a central role during normal walking. The description of the pelvic movement starts from a neutral position (the so-

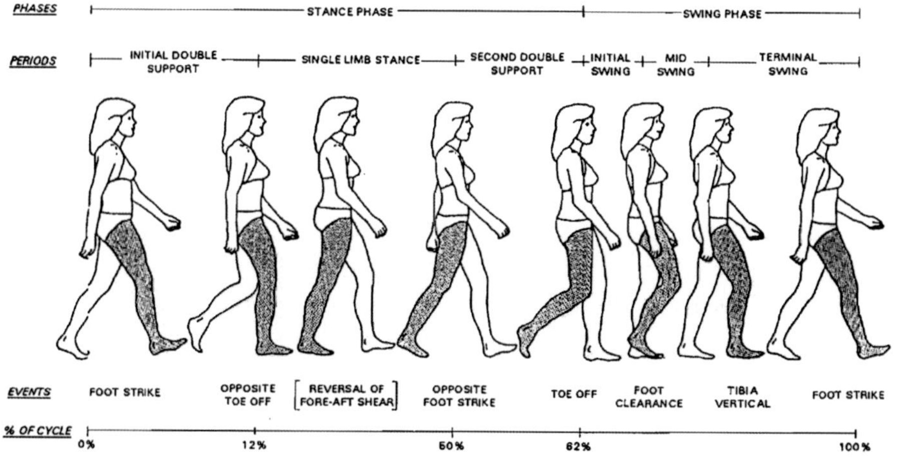

Figure 2.2: Normal gait cycle illustrating the events of gait extracted from [89].

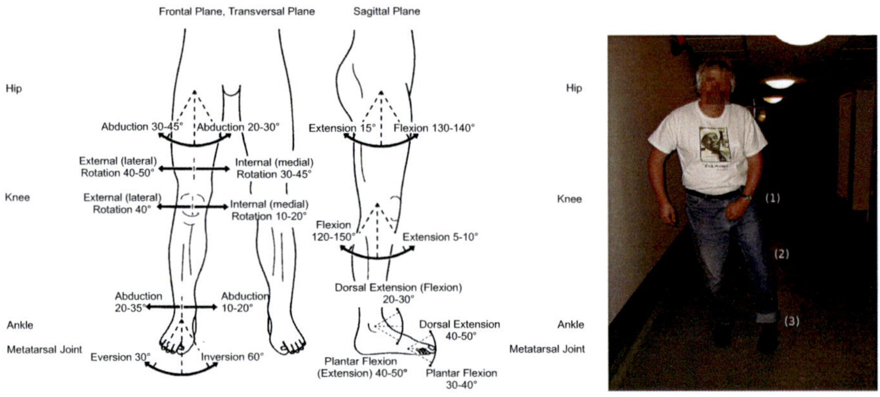

(a) (b)

Figure 2.3: (a) Movement Range of Lower Body Limbs adapted from [104]. (b) A patient with a left sided hemiparesis showing a pathologic *flexion synergy* pattern on the impaired side (property of Department for neurological rehabilitation, Charité Berlin).

called *neutral-null position*) where the pelvic tilt[1] is about 10°. The pelvic obliquity[2] and the pelvic rotation[3] are 0°. During gait cycle the pelvis shows a three-dimensional movement. The pelvis rotates with respect to the vertical axis for about $\pm5°$ during normal walking whose extent increases with the stride length. Beside the pelvis rotation in the transverse plane, the pelvic obliquity of about 4°-7° and the pelvic tilt of about 4° happen during gait. These rotations nearly completely compensate the vertical COM movement to about average 2.5cm [75].

On account of the weight takeover of one leg to the other it comes to a lateral movement and appears to be sinusoidal while tending to the supporting leg with a maximum deflection from left to right of 4.5cm. The maximum lateral amplitude is reached at the end of the *mid stance* phase at 31% of the gait cycle [71]. The legs and feet as lower body limbs form the remaining part of the locomotor. For even ground walking the movement range of the lower body limbs are shown in figure 2.3(a). It shows that the main movements of the legs and feet are in the sagittal plane. The translational and rotational movements of the foot in the frontal and the transverse plane are small in relation to the movements in sagittal plane [75], [104]. After this introduction to normal human gait, in the next section the stroke specific abnormalities of gait are introduced.

[1] pelvic inclination in sagittal plane
[2] sideways inclination of pelvis (rotation in the frontal plane)
[3] rotation of the pelvis in the transverse plane

2.2.2 Stroke Specific Gait Abnormalities

Patients after stroke show poor coordination and dysfunctional movement patterns. The not affected sound side of the body is increasingly loaded due to the limited loading capacity of the affected side.
For complex coordinated multi-joint movements such as walking, joint torques need to be appropriately coupled during the gait cycle. Subjects after stroke often fail in coupling joint torques in an appropriate way [16]. According to [103], these couplings, also called synergies, are for the lower limbs:

- the *extension synergy* coupling hip, knee and ankle extension, hip, knee and ankle adduction and
- the *flexion synergy* coupling hip, knee and ankle flexion, hip, knee, and ankle abduction.

Instability of the lower body limbs as well as significant asymmetry reduce the quality of walking. Additionally, the patients show an increased tension of the muscles (hypertonicity) which for the *extensor synergy* pattern shows ① a hip extension, an internal hip rotation and an adduction, ② knee extension and ③ an ankle inversion and plantarflexion (see figure 2.3(b)).
For the *flexion synergy* pattern it emerges to ① hip flexion, abduction and external rotation and ② knee flexion and ankle dorsal flexion and eversion. Both profiles present gait impedance factors such as altered posture, decreased functional mobility, joint pain and predisposition to contracture formation. Subjects after stroke tend to expand the *double support* phases and the *single support* phases of the supporting sound leg due to their gait insecurities or fear to fall. Hemiparetic patients show a shortened gait cycle which is not efficient any more. The most frequent causes for a changed gait pattern are a lasting shortening of muscles (Contractures), incomplete paralyses (paresis) and spastics. Common reference literature for the pathological differences with respect to normal gait are: [23], [39], [41], [64], [76], [98].

2.3 State of the Art - Systems and Approaches for Gait Parameter Determination for Clinical Gait Analysis

In the following a general overview of the different approaches for gait parameter determination is given.

There are different methods for objective and subjective analysis of human gait. The methods for gait analysis which are currently in practical use are basically founded on the works of [75], [104], [105] and with special focus on stroke patients on [41]. Though there are many methods, they can be grouped into one of the following five categories:

1. *Diagnostic Movement Inspection*: The movement inspection concentrates among other things on subjective judgment of the stability, balance ability and symmetry of movements. Systematic observations occur on the basis of rating scales. Difficulties arise due to subjective judgment and the often lacking correspondence to previous judgments (so-called *Inter*[4]- and *Intra*[5]*-Rater-Variability*). Synchronous video recordings permit a slowed down and repeated consideration of single movement details without exhaustion of the considered patient.

2. *Distance-Time-Measurement*: It is used to measure values such as step length, step width, cadence, cycle duration and walking speed. Video recordings from the lateral view permit the determination of walking speed with the time information being calculated of the camera's frame rate. These basic gait-analytical dimensions, when combined with video recordings, offer an inexpensive and reliable resource for the verification and documentation of diagnostic movement inspections.

3. *Energy Consumption*: Measurement of the efficiency of the gait by energy consumption, e. g., oxygen consumption.

4. *Kinetics*: Measurement of kinetics comprises the analysis of forces and moments acting on joints with, e. g., force plates and electromyography (EMG) measuring the muscle activity.

5. *Kinematics*: Within this category the movement is described on the base of body segments' joint angles, their speeds or accelerations. With computer-supported motion analysis systems the positions and movements of interesting body points or markers are analyzed in relation to a base co-ordinate system. Joint angles are determined in the two-dimensional or three-dimensional space.

The quality of the results of these methods is strongly related to the complexity of the method. For instance the simple *Distance-Time-Measurement* of the 2nd category stands out due to its simplicity, but has various shortcomings (features limited information, video recordings must be viewed). An example for this is the *Timed-up-and-go-Test* which is often used for evaluating the mobility after stroke.
On the other side the marker based 3D motion capturing (5th category) is characterized by its differentiated and objective results but also by its shortcomings, e. g. its price and the

[4] variance in the subjectivity of the assessment by different therapists
[5] fluctuations in the assessment by the same therapist over time (e. g., at different therapy sessions)

relatively high set-up time (approx. 20 min. to attach the markers). These two examples show very well the general problems in clinical gait analysis, i. e., on the one hand there are systems that are simple but with limited or disadvantageous information and on the other hand the systems that are too complex, expensive and/or time-consuming. This complicates a routine application of the systems in clinical practice.

Only the latter two categories provide methods that yield objective results and a distinction of the gait phases and the functional duties of the phases by considering typical joint positions and muscle activities. Since the fourth category is complex and needs a non-negligible set up time, this work focuses on the fifth category: the extraction of the kinematics.

2.3.1 Systems and Approaches for the Capturing of Human Body Kinematics

Up to now a lot of effort has been spend in the development of systems for human motion kinematics capturing. The most important systems and approaches can be classified into three main categories which differ in the location of the sensor and the source of the measured value. These categories are:

- *Inside-Out* with the sensors on the body and the sources of the measured value not on the body,
- *Inside-In* with the sensors and sources on the body and
- *Outside-In* with the sources on the body and the sensors not on the body.

The *Outside-In* category is described more in detail than the former categories because the realized approach belongs to the latter category. Therewith, the marker-based approaches are described because they form the basis for the evaluation of the realized approach.

2.3.1.1 Inside-Out Systems

Inside-Out systems are characterized by sensors that are mounted on the body while the measured value sources are not on the body. A typical representative of this category is an acoustic tracking system. Here, microphones are mounted on the body and three way speakers emit a signal whose time needed to be received by the microphones is measured. The microphones' locations on the body then are computed through triangulation.
Such a sensor measuring by means of sound is advantageous because it covers occlusions of the microphones, but conversely cables are needed. Additionally, disadvantageously

the size of the capture area is limited, sound reflections reduce accuracy and transmission rate of sound is limited.

2.3.1.2 Inside-In Systems

The *Inside-In* category features sensors and measurand source to be both directly mounted on the body. The forces and accelerations of the body directly work on the sensors (see figure 2.4(a) and (b)). The sensors can be of many different sensor types, like accelerometers, gyroscopes or goniometers which can be realized by different techniques like, e. g., electro mechanic or fiber optical systems. Inferences about posture and movement of the body are based on the knowledge about the locations of the sensors on the body and the measured data. In general, these sensors are working out their location on the base of their orientation which shows some drawbacks. Especially, accelerometers and gyroscopes fail in providing an accurate position data because acceleration data needs to be integrated twice to get position data which generally comes along with a baseline drift. Apart from this, the sensors' positions on the body must be kept constant throughout the whole measurement process. This counts also for measurements that are carried out at different times because otherwise the measuring exactness decreases. Hence, the application of these sensors lead to high set up time and the need in especially qualified staff. This prevents the application in the clinical everyday life.

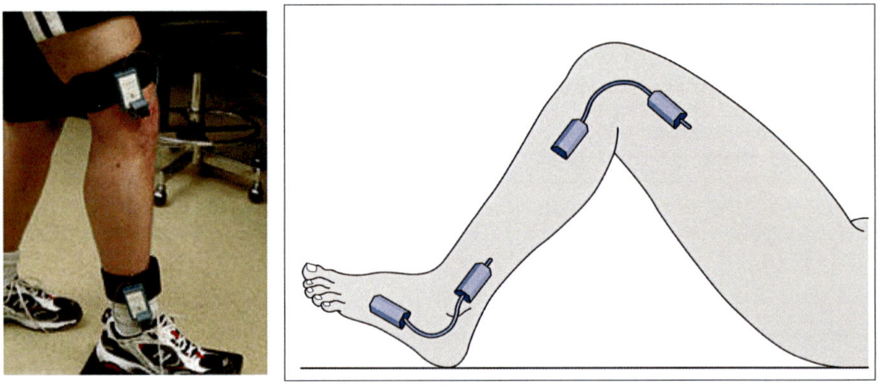

(a) (b)

Figure 2.4: (a) Subject with mounted accelerometers. (b) Subject wearing flexible goniometers on knee and ankle. Adapted from manufacturers' literature ((a) CleveMed, (b) Biometrics Ltd).

2.3.1.3 Outside-In Systems

Any system which relies on external sensors that capture the body belongs to the *Outside-In* category. In the following only the electro-optical approaches are considered because this work focuses on the optical measurement of kinematics.
Video based measurement of kinematics can be done either in 2D or in 3D. Since 2D systems just perform a projection of the 3D environment onto the 2D sensor plane, only movements on this projection plane are captured. Therefore, 2D-systems suffer from ambiguities in depth. For this reason, without any use of model information, these systems are normally only used for the measurement of joint angles such as the knee angle in the sagittal plane from a lateral view. Here, any part of the angulations which occurs out of that plane is lost. Depth approximations can be included into the measurement when using some form of calibration object like a system known calibration pattern which is placed behind the person whose movements are to be captured.
Since human body movements happen in the three dimensions and to achieve reasonable accurate kinematic measurements, measurements that aim to universally capture movements need to be realized by systems that capture all three dimensions.
There are two general approaches that can be distinguished, the marker based and the markerless approach which are briefly presented in the following because both form a central part of this work.

MARKER BASED 3D SYSTEMS
At the moment marker based systems are considered to be the 'gold standard' for human motion capturing for clinical motion analysis studies and are generally realized as multi-camera systems with 6-12 cameras in the majority of cases. The main idea of marker based systems is to track markers which are mounted on a subject and to determine the position of these markers in 3D space over time. The joint positions are computed based on the positions of these markers which are either active (self illuminating) such as light emitting diodes (LED) or passive such as reflective or specially colored markers. Passive markers are somewhat more practical because power supply is not needed. A subject with attached reflective markers is shown in figure 2.5(a). To determine the position of the markers in the 3D space, triangulation is applied which requires the markers to be seen at all frames by at least two cameras with known camera pose. Triangulation is used to determine the position in 3D. In figure 2.5(b) a measurement scene with eight cameras for marker tracking is shown. The set up is designed in a redundant manner with eight cameras to cope with occlusions of markers.

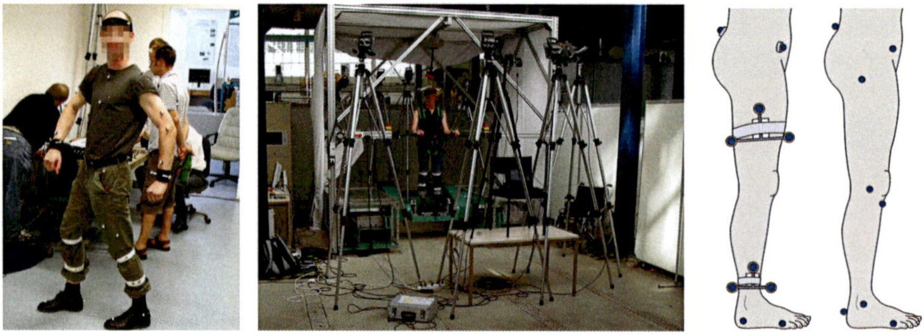

(a) (b) (c)

Figure 2.5: (a) A person with mounted markers. (b) A measurement setup for human kinematics capturing with the *IR*-cameras of the marker based system encircling the marker equipped person in the *HapticWalker*. (c) Two examples of marker sets, *left* with a rigid structure and *right* with markers placed at anatomical landmarks, extracted from [104].

The placement of the markers on the body can be carried out in different ways which can be divided into two fundamentally different approaches. One method is characterized by placing the markers directly on the skin at anatomical landmarks which are defined by the used marker set. The other approach comprises in attaching rigid sets of at least three markers to each limb segment. This can be done either directly or with a rigid structure the markers are attached on. The position and orientation of the rigid structure can be determined in 3D space. The position of the joint center is computed out of this. Figure 2.5(c) visualizes these two ways to arrange markers for the lower limbs by mounting markers on a rigid structure (left) or at anatomical landmarks (right). The marker based motion capture system that is used for the evaluation of the developed method establishes the latter method which is the most common method.

For markers' placement there are some schemes which essentially are variants of the *Conventional Gait Model*. In this thesis the *Plug-In Gait* marker set is employed for evaluation because it is one of the most common marker sets. One has to keep in mind that these marker sets, although being used for evaluation of the developed system, may not be satisfactorily good for patients due to possible dysplasia [3]. Nevertheless, this is not in focus of this work.

Current marker based systems provide an accuracy of less than $1mm$ in sense of measurement inherent errors [101]. Further errors mainly originate from non-static positioned markers during the measurements. This is due to, e. g., skin movement relative to the underlying bone or joint, respectively. These errors are subsumed as *soft tissue artifacts*, e. g., Roux et. al. [90] who determines the error due to skin movement to be up to $3cm$ if markers are placed at unfavorable positions. Leardinia et. al. [56] determines the worst case mean square error to be 7° for bone orientation. Though these systems are the 'gold standard' they have several further limitations which strengthen the need for markerless systems as considered within this work. These limitations are listed in the overview table 2.1 at page 16.

MARKERLESS 3D SYSTEMS

Markerless systems waive the usage of markers for posture determination. Some research work has been done in the field of markerless 3D systems for clinical gait analysis purpose. These systems are realized in the majority of cases by multi-camera approaches with known camera poses. Most of them perform volume carving through a projection of the silhouette into 3D space *Shape from Silhouette (SfS)* (see 2.4.1). But satisfactory results for applicability in clinical gait analysis have not been accomplished up to now [3]. Other approaches also work with multiple cameras but rather as multiple combined 2D-systems with different projection planes. Only one approach is based on a depth camera, but in comparison to this work with a different purpose.

Since the development of a markerless system is the main objective of this work, the most related works for 3D markerless optical human kinematics measurement for the purpose of gait analysis are reviewed in detail in the sections 2.3.2. The focus, thereby, is set on different sensory bases.

2.3.1.4 Overview - Systems for Human Kinematics Capturing

The objective of this section is to provide an overview of the aforementioned approaches which highlights their advantages and disadvantages in a comparable way (see table 2.1).

MOTION CAPTURE SYSTEM	ADVANTAGES	DISADVANTAGES
Inside-Out	• handles marker occlusion (acoustic)	• limited capture volume • prone to multi reflections (acoustic) • set-up time • alter movements
Inside-In	• low requirement on environment	• set-up time • relative data (no position data) • alter movements • sensor weight might increase soft tissue artifact
Outside-In, marker based	• data accuracy ($\leq$ 1mm, [101])	• costs as limiting factor for most laboratories • limited capture volume that must be calibrated beforehand • set-up time for accurate marker placement ($\approx$ 20 min.) • limited repeatability due to inappropriate model set, inaccurate marker placement, model calibration, soft tissue artifacts, etc. ($\leq$ 3cm, [90], $\leq$ 2cm,[31]) • prone to marker occlusion • alter movements
Outside-In markerless	• set-up time • do not alter movements	• limited capture volume • accuracy • prone to occlusions

Table 2.1: This table provides an overview over the different motion capture system approaches and their advantages and disadvantages.

2.3.2 Research Activities for 3D Markerless Optical Motion Capture for Gait Analysis

In the following some of the most related research activities in the field of human motion tracking for the purpose of gait parameter estimation are presented. Thereby, different sensory approaches are selected.

2.3.2.1 BioMotion Research Group of Stanford Mechanical Engineering Department

One of the most active research groups working in the field of markerless motion capture for the purpose of performing gait analysis is the *BioMotion* research group of the *Stanford University*. The main target of this group is to study normal and pathological gait function for the improved evaluation and treatment of musculoskeletal disease and injury. Besides this, the BioMotion group aims to improve methods for the capturing and analysis of human motion without any markers. The main motivation of this group is to realize an alternative to marker based systems which is less expensive, reduces the set-up time, does not alter the movements of the tracked person and yields accurate measurement results. These goals equate to the goals pursued within this work. But moreover, in this work a non-complex system with small space requirement is pursued and which copes with the bars and supporting harness of the demonstrator scenario.

The system is established on a multi-2D-camera-approach applying *shape-from-silhouette* (SfS) [19]. As one of the most widespread approaches for human motion capture, it will

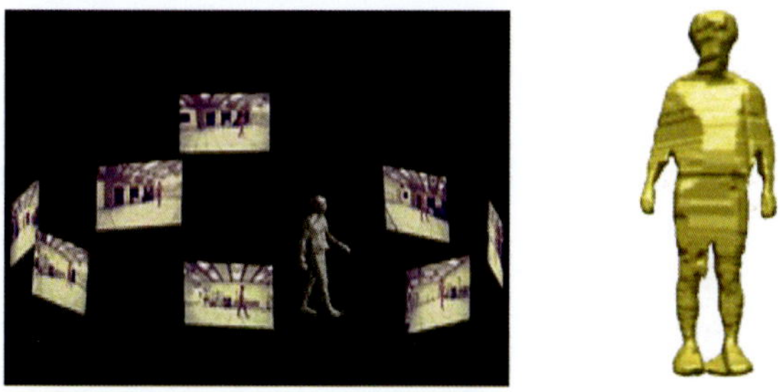

(a) (b)

Figure 2.6: (a) shows a multi-camera-approach applying *Shape-from-Silhouette* which was followed by the BioMotion research group of the Stanford university. The performance of this approach is dependent on the number and positions of the surrounding cameras. (b) a volume which was carved out of the 3D capture volume by reprojecting the 2D-silhouettes of the person from every single camera. The lines of sight from each camera defined by the objects' silhouettes can clearly be identified and result in the polygonal appearance of the volume.

be described in section 2.4.1. In summary, SfS projects the 2D silhouettes of the tracked object (i. e., the person) into 3D and carves out the object in 3D. The figure 2.6(a) shows the cameras positioned around the person and capturing the person walking within the field of view (FOV) of the surrounding cameras. This directly reveals the major drawback of this approach which is the systems' complexity and space requirement. Therefore, the ToF range imaging camera approach was chosen in this work. Furthermore, the SfS-approach needs an unobstructed view for all cameras. This is not given for considered demonstrator scenario. Another short-coming of this approach is that it is prone to concave objects as is the human body to a very high degree. It performs best for convex objects. To compensate for these deficits to some extent the number of different views is normally increased. An essay on the effect of the number of cameras on the accuracy of the data is given in section 2.4.1 which shows that 8 cameras result in a volumetric error of $\approx 15\%$. Nevertheless, this does not remedy the problem with concave surfaces. Here, additional approaches have to be applied to estimate the real surface characteristics, e. g. *Shape-from-Texture* [48], *Shape-from-Shading* [107] or by using the TOF camera instead. In figure 2.6(b) the carved out volume is shown. The lines of sight from each camera defined by the silhouettes can clearly be identified and result in the polygonal appearance of the volume. One critical aspect of the development of biomechanical analysis systems is the measurement of internal-external rotation of the pelvis, hip and the knee. The chosen approach of 3D model fitting into a 3D volume is limited in capturing such movements due to the cylindrical symmetry of the thigh and shank. At the moment this represents the main limitation of the approach. As will be seen later in this work this issue is faced with temporally tracked corners (e. g., SURF [5]) on the body.

The presented system captures the scene with a frame rate of $200Hz$. It may be pointed out that the range imaging camera used in our system is working at a frame rate of $30Hz$ which results in a bigger difference between two images when capturing an object with the same motion. This especially affects the tracking procedure since bigger changes result in a bigger search space.

According to the BioMotion group the system is providing sufficient accuracy for biomechanical research. The accuracy of the system was demonstrated experimentally. A comparison / validation against current available techniques such as marker based methods like the *Vicon*® system [101] used in this work is pending and marked as future work. Future improvements of the system lie in the creation of the model and in the matching algorithm. The processing frame rate achieved with this system is not stated exactly. As a rough impression the processing for a short test sequence of a person running across the measurement track is stated to last a few hours.

2.3.2.2 Institut für Elektronik, Signalverarbeitung und Kommunikationstechnik, Otto-von-Guericke-Universität Magdeburg

The 'Institut für Elektronik, Signalverarbeitung und Kommunikationstechnik' (IESK) at the Otto-von-Guericke-Universität in Magdeburg approaches the motion capturing of human gait with a multi-2D-camera system. The figure 2.7(a) shows the setup of the cameras along the measurement track. In contrast to the work of the Stanford BioMotion group which uses the *SfS*-method and match a 3D-model into the 3D volume, here, a 2D-model is matched into every single camera view image which correspond either the sagittal or the frontal perspective. This means that it has to be guaranteed that the gait movements occur according to these perspectives. This forms a major limitation of this approach. The main idea is to match a 2D-model into the images of the cameras surrounding the track. On the base of the information of all 2D matches, afterwards a 3D-model is fit into the 2D matches. Thereby, a movement model is used which describes the cyclic gait with Fourier descriptors. Another concern of this system is the automated adaption of the system to a subject with a coarse manual initialization of the model.

The difficulty of this approach lies in the fact that difficult situations have to be solved for every single image like, e. g., when the legs are crossed during swing phase from the side view which is displayed in figure 2.7(b). On the base of the displayed single image it is first attempted to detect the occlusion. Afterwards the silhouettes of the occluded lower limbs are estimated. The recovered silhouettes of the lower limbs are matched to

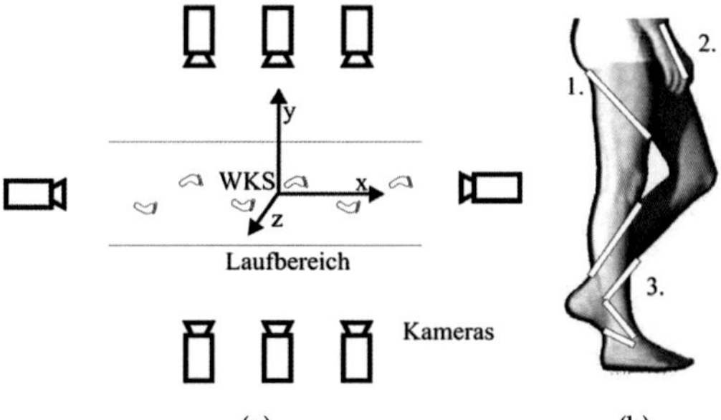

Figure 2.7: (a) shows the multi-camera system setup of the *IESK*. (b) is an image of a camera on the side of the measurement track. The image shows a person with one leg occluding the other when passing the camera. From this single image the occlusion first is tried to detect. Then the silhouettes of the occluded lower body limb are estimated. As a model for the silhouettes of the lower limbs simple straight lines are applied [17].

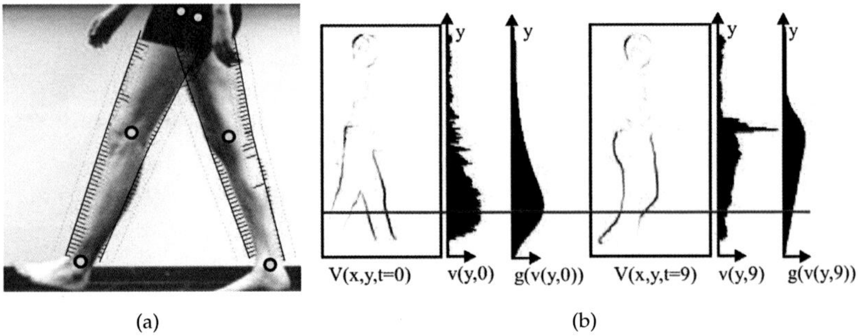

Figure 2.8: (a) Approximation of the model with corresponding joints. (b) Line-by-line motion variance for the double-support phase on the left and the single-stance-phase on the right [17].

the 2D-shape model for each camera view. The information of the other cameras is not exploited at this stage of the procedure.

The figure 2.8(a) shows a projection of the 2D-model of the shank and the thigh of both legs from the side view. Before that the gross motion of the body is estimated through computation of a line-by-line motion integral which gives an idea about the current gait phase and enables the system to automatically initialize the model. The figure 2.8(b) illustrates this. Here, the red line represents an example of a horizontal line along which the motion is summed up. For motion determination a frame-by-frame subtraction is carried out. The line-by-line motion values are displayed beside the images. This information is then taken for further posture refinement on the base of cyclic gait models. As one can directly imagine this step assumes the person to walk upright and the cameras to be oriented horizontally.

The approach showed that it is capable to determine the joint angle curves of the hip and the knee accurate and reproducible. Well determined is the translational motion in x-and z-direction. A moderate accuracy in the determination of the ankle joint angle was achieved. Even less reproducibility was achieved for the capture of the leg abduction and adduction. As cause the normal biological variability of the gait is given. As with any measurement system uncertainties remain with the parameter settings.

2.3.2.3 IMM, Technical University of Denmark

The only work which is also based on TOF camera data is that of Jensen et. al. [43]. In the work the sagittal plane of a subject walking on a treadmill is captured from the side. The aim of this work is to estimate the temporal-spatial gait parameters, such as the step length by estimating the initial heel contact and the toe off of both feet, the cadence, the

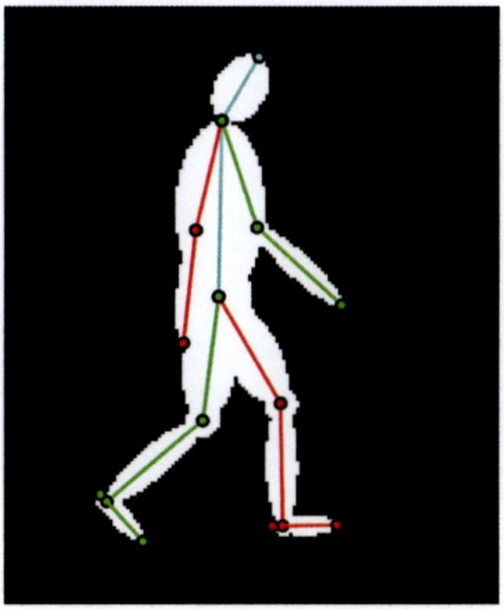

Figure 2.9: 2D stick model used in the work of [43] which is fitted into a 2D foreground object estimate. The foreground segmentation is gained by exploiting the depth data.

speed and the joint angles of the sagittal plane. They employ an adapted version of pose cut which includes depth data as well as intensity data and synthesizes the posture about a 2D stick model with the help of markov random field.

The depth data in this work is solely used for the foreground background segmentation. Thereby, the background is statistically modeled. That means that the mean μ_b and the standard deviation σ_b are computed for every pixel for a few frames without any foreground object. The segmentation of the foreground is achieved by comparing the background data set (μ_b, σ_b) with the mean μ and standard deviation σ of that moment for each pixel. The determination of the joint angles is performed on the base of this foreground data.
The approach assumes that the TOF camera is aligned perpendicular to the sagittal plane of the subject. Because the angles are only determined with respect to the perpendicular positioned camera, the approach does not extract all relevant gait parameters and, therefore, is not adequate for gait analysis. The work provides a method for automated initialization of the 2D-stick model which seems to perform well. Objective information about the performance of the presented method is not given so that an evaluation of the results with reference data is pending. The comparison of the results with a marker based system is pending. Because a 2D stick model is used which is generated beforehand for the to-be-analyzed gait pattern, this approach might suppress the pathologic as well as the individual characteristics of gait patterns and, thus, not sensitive enough for this purpose. Therefore, this approach seems not appropriate for the concerns aimed in this work. Additionally, this work just focuses on the temporal-spatial parameters that are given by the rehabilitation robot used in this work which focuses on the determination

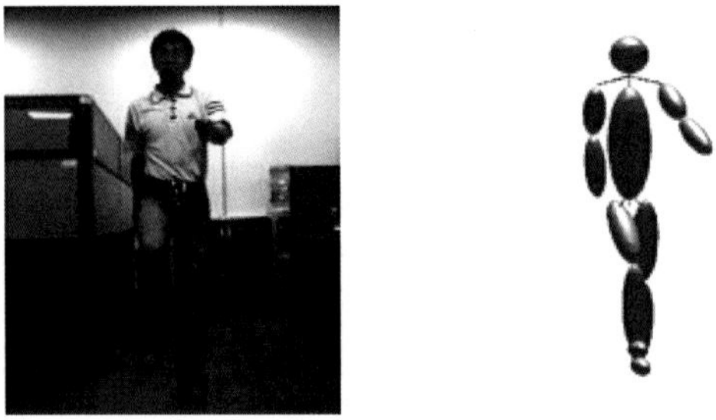

(a) (b)

Figure 2.10: (a) one image of the used stereo vision system. (b) shows the rendered ellipsoid-model that synthesizes the posture of the person in image (a) [72].

of gait traces. Nevertheless, this work represents an interesting approach with potential, although it is believed that the in advance learned cyclic model is not suited to determine individual pathologic characteristics.

2.3.2.4 Department of Biomedical Engineering, Kyung Hee University, South Korea

This work is also based on depth data, but the depth data is acquired with a stereo vision system. Like all the other presented research activities, this method is also model-based. The model consists of rigid ellipsoids that represent the respective body segments. These ellipsoids are connected by a kinematic chain. The depth data of this algorithm is reprojected into the 3D space, as it is performed in the realized system of this work. These 3D points are assigned to the segments of the human body model on the base of the Euclidean distance between each 3D point to each body segment. A 3D point is assigned to the ellipsoid which is nearest from the 3D point. Thereby, methods are used to detect the face and the torso in the images to provide extra information for the assignment. Additionally, to avoid an incorrect assignment, geodesic constraints are applied which incorporates a smoothing term. The posture is synthesized by minimizing the distances between 3D point and the model on a frame-by-frame basis. That means that the current model fitting process is initialized by the posture synthesis of the previously synthesized posture. This is performed by using a least square optimization.
An objective evaluation of the performance of the algorithm is not performed. The figure 2.10 represents an example of the results that are given. Therefore, a statement about the performance of the algorithm cannot be given. Due the use of a stereo vision system the system is non-complex, but on the other hand shows the systematic deficit of stereo vision for convex objects (see figure 2.14). Furthermore, stereo vision needs correspondences which are often not present on cloth.

2.3.2.5 ECS, University of Southampton (UK)

The ECS approaches the extraction of gait parameters with a single 2D-camera and, therefore, completely do without depth information. This forms a major shortcoming of the work.
ECS activities are centered in fundamental theory and algorithm development associated with many engineering areas amongst others the biomechanical field. Within the ISIS research group at the Department of Electronics and Computer Science at the University of Southampton the *DARPA* funded program 'Automatic Gait Recognition for Human ID at a Distance' a markerless system was developed which is based on a single view 2D-camera. This program concerns developing new technologies for recognizing people at a distance. One major aim of the project was to develop a database for research work in automatic gait recognition. The proposed approach for gait recognition is based on moving-feature extraction and description techniques. One major drawback of this approach is that due to the single camera approach the depth information is lost. References about the accuracy and the processing time of the system are not given [32]. However, without incorporating the third dimension the accuracy of the system is limited. The idea of the proposed work is to estimate the view angle $\mu[^\circ]$ of a person. The figure 2.11 shows some examples of two different view angles $\mu = 0^\circ$ and $\mu = 20^\circ$. For the view angle $\mu = 0^\circ$ different gait phases are shown and exemplary demonstrating the robustness. Experimental tests have been conducted on about two hundred video sequences. Three persons were viewed at six different camera view angles. Nevertheless, this approach, although focusing on the analysis of gait parameters, seems to be limited when complex movements occur.

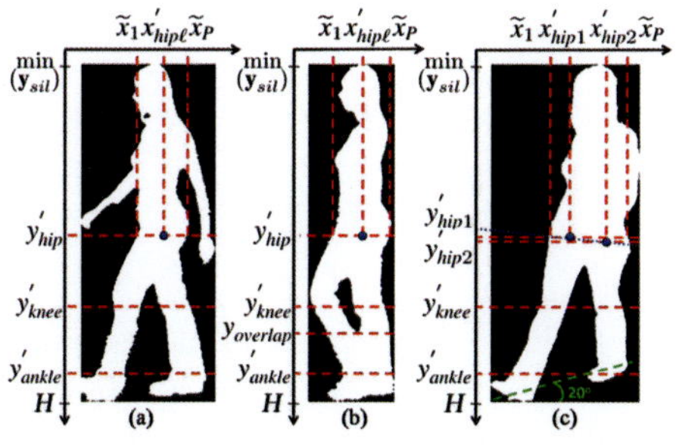

Figure 2.11: Some examples of the estimation of the view angle μ a person is looked at. (a) $\mu = 0^\circ$ view with no overlapping and (b) with overlapping feet; (c) $\mu = 20^\circ$ view.

2.4 State of the Art - Time-of-Flight Range Imaging Cameras

Because a sensor forms the base of the realized system, the different sensors need to be balanced with respect to the considered task. Therefore, the different sensors are presented. But when talking about sensors one also has to talk about the different sensor data types which are provided by the sensors. For this reason a brief definition of the different types of sensor data (2D-$2\frac{1}{2}$D-3D) and the related sensor principles is given before we step over to the state of the art of TOF Range Imaging Cameras.

2.4.1 2D - $2\frac{1}{2}$D - 3D Sensor Data and Sensor Principles

2D - SENSOR DATA AND PRINCIPLES

2D data normally refers to a two dimensional projection of a 3D scene such that one dimension, normally the depth, is neglected. In contrast laser range scanners neglect either the height or the width but always keep the depth. In the following 2D refers to the first interpretation of 2D.

$2\frac{1}{2}$D - SENSOR DATA AND PRINCIPLES

$2\frac{1}{2}$D data is characterized by the depth between the sensor system and the objects of the scene with regard to sensor systems field of view (FOV). This is in contrast to 2D-cameras sensors which capture the luminance or chrominance, respectively. For this reason $2\frac{1}{2}$D data is also called depth data. An example of depth data and 2D data is shown in figure 2.12. In the last decades a number of different sensor principles to capture $2\frac{1}{2}$D data had been developed which are shortly introduced in the following.

TIME-OF-FLIGHT

Sensors working on the base of Time-of-Flight (TOF) generally measure the time of the emitted light reflected by the object of a captured scene. Since this type of sensor forms the sensor base of this work it will be explained in detail in the section 2.4.3.

STEREOSCOPY[6] (STEREO VISION)

The stereoscopic principle is a fairly old principle which is actually the principle of the human vision system. The main idea behind it is the correspondence analysis of images taken from at least two spatially different camera views. The different camera views can be captured at a single time step with different cameras or sequentially with one moving camera. In the latter case it is called *structure-from-motion* which becomes a demanding task when the object is moving. On the other hand this approach is not restricted to

[6]Originally Greek with *stereo* 'spatial' and *skopeia* 'consideration'

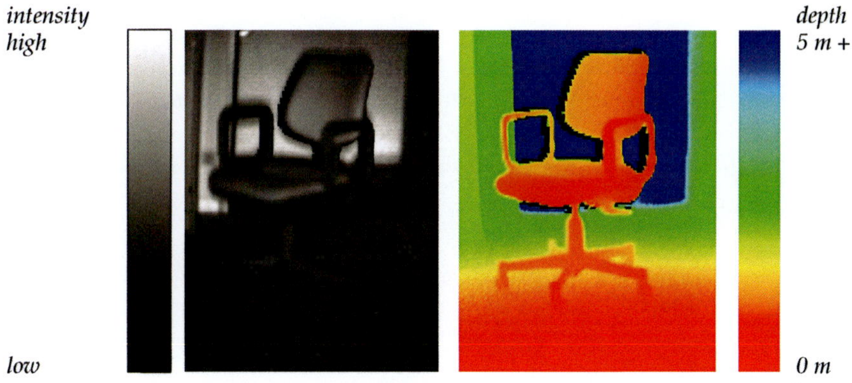

Figure 2.12: *left:* The 2D intensity image of a scene. *right:* The corresponding $2\frac{1}{2}$D data of the same scene. The depth is color coded according the legend on the right.

any fixed transformation between the sensors. In stereo vision the depth is calculated of the known transformation between the camera views in conjunction with the correspondences between the different images. The theoretical base is the epipolar geometry which describes the projective relations between pixels of the images captured from the different views (see figure 2.13) [29]. To understand the advantages and disadvantages of stereo vision, especially in contrast to TOF-sensors which form the base of this work, the theoretical base is briefly explained.

In the figure 2.13 the 3D-point P is projected onto the sensor plane to P_1 and P_2 according to the camera projection centers C_1 and C_2 of the two considered cameras. The plane defined by P, C_1 and C_2 is called the epipolar plane. It defines the epipolar line of both cameras by the intersection their sensor planes. The benefit of the epipolar line is that it describes the search space for finding the corresponding points in the two images (in this case $P_1 \Leftrightarrow P_2$). This requires the points to be characteristic enough in their neighborhood

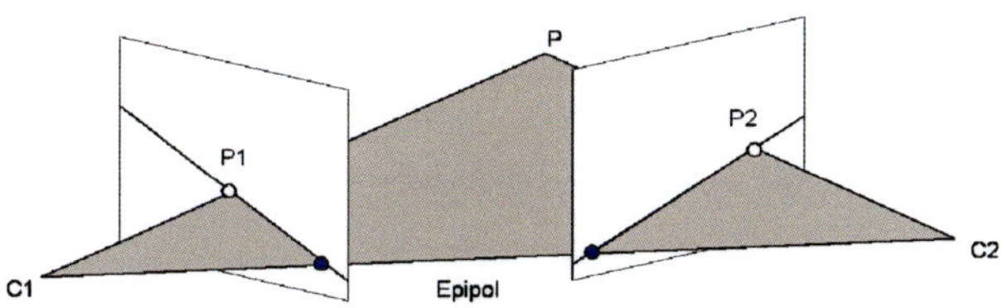

Figure 2.13: Epipolar geometry of two cameras which project the 3D-point P of the scene through the projection centers C_1 and C_2 onto P_1 and P_2 in the sensor plane. The so-called epipols are drawn in blue.

to be not mistaken with other points and at the same time to be similar enough from the considered views to be correctly assigned to each other. This requirement forms the main limitation of this approach. *Stereo vision*, therefore, needs structures. These are normally edges between different objects or textures. Since the limbs of a human are convex, the correspondence analysis in this case suffers from a systematic error in the depth measurement D_{error} which is dependent on the base distance b between the two considered views, the limb curvature r and the distance to the limb edge D (see figure 2.14). On the base of an angle error β_{error} and distance error D_{error} with $\Delta d = r \cdot tan\frac{\alpha}{2}$ results to:

$$\begin{aligned} \beta_{error} &= \arctan \frac{\Delta d \cdot sin\alpha}{D - \Delta d(1 + cos\alpha)} \\ D_{error} &= \Delta d(1 + cos\alpha) \end{aligned} \tag{2.1}$$

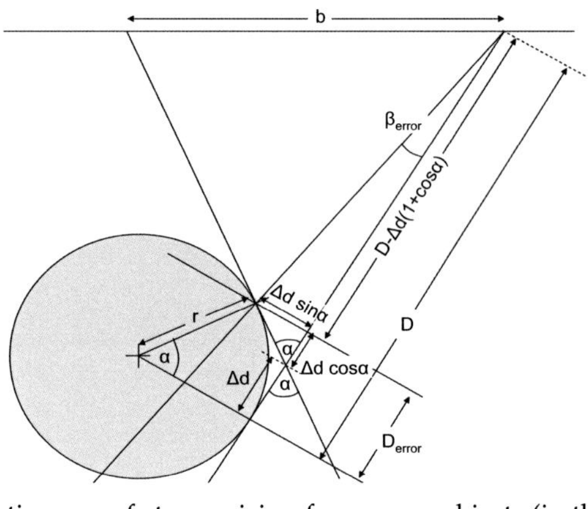

Figure 2.14: Systematic error of stereo vision for convex objects (in this case for simplification with a circular curvature) (see text for parameters).

3D - SENSOR DATA AND PRINCIPLES

3D sensor data completely captures all three spatial dimensions. The 3D-capturing of human bodies is normally established on the base of a combined capture of 2D- and/or $2\frac{1}{2}$D data, respectively, to avoid the use of unhealthy radiation such as x-rays. The most popular approach used for human movement capturing is *shape-from-silhouette* (SfS). Therefore it is explained in the following.

SHAPE-FROM-SILHOUETTE (SfS)

SfS which is also called *shape-from-contour* was first introduced by [63] and [33]. It is a multi-camera approach which captures the objects from different views. Foreground segmentation for every camera yields the silhouette of the considered object from each cam-

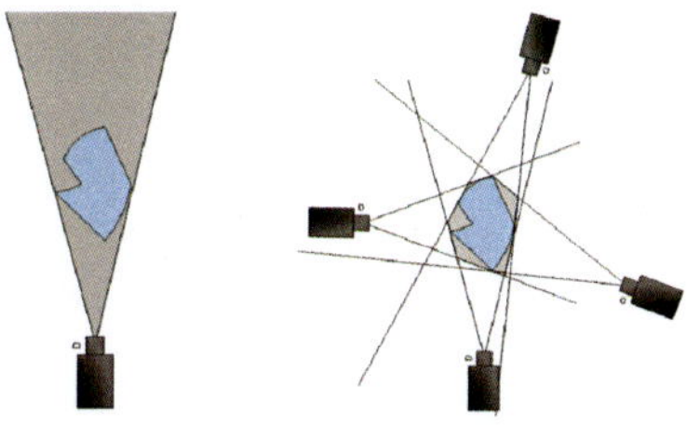

(a) (b)

Figure 2.15: (a) When reprojecting the silhouette of an object into 3D, a volume is defined (the gray area). With just one view this volume represents a very coarse approximation cv_{obj} of the geometry $real_{obj}$ (the blue area) which is refined by incorporating additional variant views (b).

eras' view. When projecting the 2D-silhouettes into 3D, a projection volume is defined which is called a *truncated extended silhouette*. The considered object with the geometry $real_{obj}$ lies within this volume. An example for this is shown in figure 2.15 (a). If intersection this volume with the volumes generated from the other cameras' views, a volume cv_{obj} results which is called the *convex hull*. It approximates the geometry $real_{obj}$. The more different views are used for volume generation, the better the *convex hull* approximates the $real_{obj}$ (see figure 2.15 (b)). This converges to the smallest possible volume, the *visual hull* (vh_{obj}). If and only if the considered object is convex, the volumes vh_{obj} and $real_{obj}$ theoretically can become identical. When the object is concave, vh_{obj} and $real_{obj}$ cannot become identical. This can be expressed with the following equation.

$$real_{obj} \subseteq vh_{obj} \subseteq ch_{obj} \tag{2.2}$$

Generally spoken, the quality of the volume reconstructed by *SfS* is prone to errors due to occlusions, concave objects or the lack of appropriate camera views. Figure 2.16 demonstrates the strong dependency of the *SfS*-approach on the number of cameras.

Additionally, the necessity of different camera views raises the overall system complexity, which makes this approach spacious and, therefore, only in a limited way feasible for clinical gait analysis. For future applications such as home treatment SfS is not suited.
The most important error sources of SfS are according to [73]:

- Correctness of the camera parameters, i. e., a precise camera calibration.
- Quantization error of the silhouette.
- Quantization error of the volume which is normally adapted according to the applications requirements, e. g., run-time, accuracy, etc..

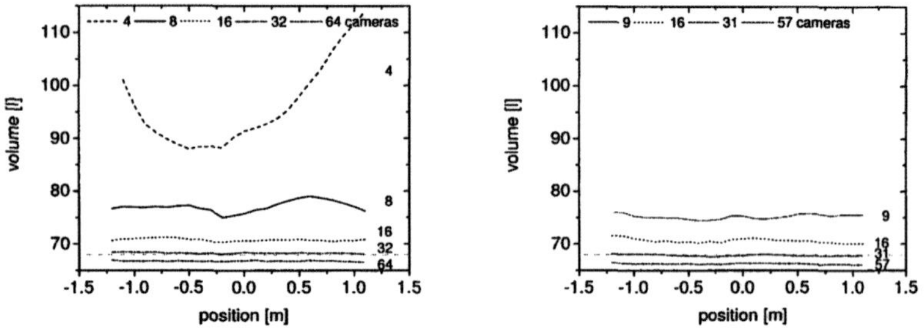

Figure 2.16: *'Visual hull'* vh_{obj} as a function of the number of cameras and their positions for a walking person with a volume of about 68 liters. The plot on the left shows the results for a circular and uniform distribution of the cameras at a height of $1m$. An additional camera is placed above the head. On the right side the results for a hemispherical uniform distribution are plotted. Both plots are extracted from [68].

- Number and orientation of different views according to convexity/concavity of the object.

2.4.1.1 Overview - Sensors and Sensor data types

The table 2.2 shows a matrix of the different approaches applicable in human movement capturing with respect to the spatial dimension of the sensor data provided by the sensor system and the sensor principles.

2.4.2 Time-of-Flight Range Imaging Cameras

As already mentioned, the sensory basis for this work is a TOF range imaging sensor. Because 'out-of-the-box' the sensor is not ready for gait parameter extraction, a data enhancement step has to be carried out at first. But due to the novelty of this kind of sensor and the absence of appropriate enhancement methods, according methods had to be developed. Therefore, this section is about the development of data enhancement methods which significantly reduces the distance offset and, hence, allows the use of the chosen TOF range imaging sensor for our purpose.
During the works of this dissertation, the sensors had been evolved significantly, i. e., achieving an increase in the frame rate (as well as in its constancy) and in the lateral resolution. This led to the decision to undergo a change to a newer sensor, so that during this work we switched from the depth camera *PMD [vision] 19k* that was used at the starting time, to the *3DVSystems ZCam*. Pictures of these cameras are presented in figure 2.17. Another important characteristic of the *ZCam* is the combined active and passive illumi-

sensor data

sensor principle	2D	2,5D	3D
2D	• *2D Camera*	• *2D - Stereo* • *Structure from Motion / Stereo*	• *2D - Shape from Silhouette*
2,5D		• *2,5D - Stereo* • *Time-of-Flight (ToF)*	• *2,5D - Shape from Silhouette*
3D			

Table 2.2: Combinations of sensor principles and sensor data regarding their spatial dimension with exemplary approches relevant to this work.

nation concept which leads to a separability of some distance error sources and yields a more stable depth calibration as will be seen in the related section later on. Nevertheless, the work to improve the *PMD [vision] 19k*-data represents important preliminary work and, therefore, is also presented in this dissertation.

In the following the principles of the both range imaging cameras are presented. This is followed by the error sources and there improvements, i. e., the calibration of the data retrieved from the cameras.

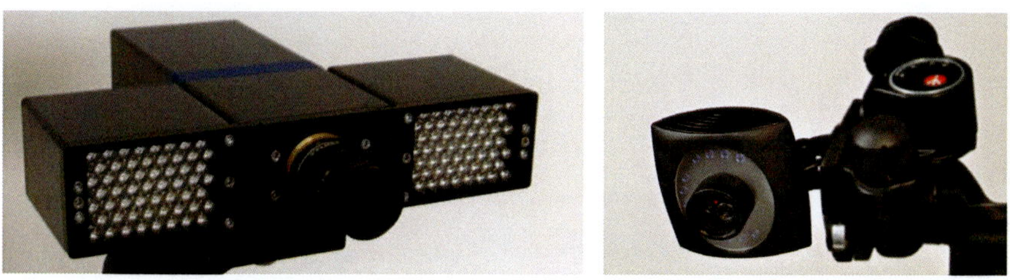

(a) (b)

Figure 2.17: (a) The *PMD [vision] 19k* and (b) the *3DVSystems ZCam*.

2.4.3 Principles of Time-of-Flight Range Imaging Cameras

Within this section the principles of the two used TOF range imaging cameras are presented. Since both cameras rely on a different principle each camera is given a proper section.

2.4.3.1 Principles of *PMD [vision] 19k*

To measure the distance range imaging cameras apply the Time-of-Flight principle whose main idea is to measure the time which is needed by an emitted light signal to get back and forth to an object. The *PMD [vision] 19k* achieves this by directly sampling and correlating the reflected signal with the emitted reference signal on the chip. Thereby, the depth information d is determined by the signal's phase shift φ between incoming signal and the reference signal. See the following equation 2.3 for distance calculation.

$$d = \frac{\varphi \cdot c}{4\pi \cdot f} \tag{2.3}$$

Here, c is the speed of light and f the fixed frequency the signals are modulated with. From the correlation function CF the basic parameters can be extracted: the modulation amplitude $Ampl$ and the phase shift φ. φ is then calculated based on the four sampling points A_1, A_2, A_3 and A_4 of the correlation function, as shown in equation 2.5. See equation 2.4 for sampling point calculation.

$$A_i = CF(\frac{\pi}{2} \cdot i) \; for \; i = 0..3 \tag{2.4}$$

$$\varphi = \arctan \frac{A_0 - A_2}{A_1 - A_3} \tag{2.5}$$

The amplitude $Ampl$ can be calculated with following equation 2.6:

$$Ampl = \frac{\sqrt{(A_0 - A_2)^2 + (A_1 - A_3)^2}}{2} \tag{2.6}$$

In [55] [62] a detailed description of the function of the PMD range imaging camera is given. In practice the accuracy differs from theory so that related errors have to be calibrated out for the use of the PMD range imaging camera. To get an overview of the most important known error sources see section 2.4.4.

2.4.3.2 Principles of the *3DVSystems ZCam*

In contrast to the *PMD [vision] 19k* for the purpose of measuring the depth, a *light pulse* with a defined width is emitted by the camera. After a fixed time the shutter is closed. Due to this fixed shutter speed, the amount of light corresponds to the depth, such that the more illuminated the pixels are, the closer the related object is. This operation is depicted

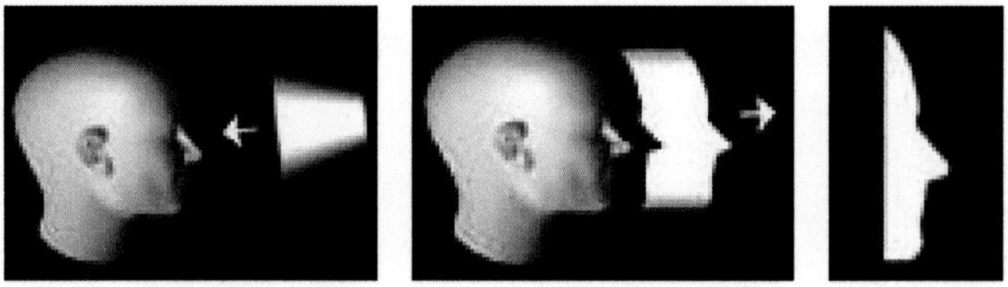

(a) (b) (c)

Figure 2.18: Operation of the TOF camera *'ZCam'* extracted from [35]. The generated and emitted light pulse (a) is reflected by the object showing an imprint of the object's frontal surface (b). By fast image shutter the reflected light pulse is cropped so that it represents an elevation profile of the object (c).

in figure 2.18.

The generated and emitted light pulse (a) is reflected by the object showing an imprint of the object's frontal surface (b). By applying a fast image shutter the reflected light pulse is cropped so that the imprint of the interesting object is frozen (c). The depth imprint is inversely proportional to the depth so that the amount of the incident light is higher when the object is closer to the camera. The following equation describes the computation of the depth d on the base of the depth value d_{val} of the depth image. The value d_{max} corresponds to the maximum 8 bit data representation, i. e., 255. The value *Dist* refers to the minimum considered distance, i. e., all objects closer than this min. distance will appear at this distance. The value *Width* is the width of the considered depth, i. e., the width of the light pulse.

$$d = Dist + Width \cdot (1 - \frac{d_{val}}{d_{max}}) \tag{2.7}$$

In [35] a detailed description of the operation of the range imaging camera *ZCam* is given. The light pulse is generated with an illumination of infra-red (IR) bandwidth.

2.4.4 Systematic errors of TOF Range Imaging Cameras

This section gives an overview over the known error sources. The taxonomy of this overview reflects the causes of the different error types and therefore depicts which errors can be handled separately. Considering the known error sources yields four major systematic errors: Error due to the inharmonic properties of the signals, the pixel-wise offset, the amount of incident light and motion. The latter systematic error due to motion exclusively occurs with motion whereas the former three always occur. A quick overview of these error sources and an estimation of their effect on the distance measurement giving the corresponding reference of this estimation is listed up in table 2.3.

EFFECT	ERROR ESTIMATE
Inharmonic properties of signals [86]	80 mm
Pixel-wise offset [86]	20 mm
Amount of incident light	
▷ due to integration time [87]	35 mm
▷ due to integration time, distance and reflectivity [58]	50-180 mm

Table 2.3: Impact estimates of different error sources on depth measurement with corresponding reference by investigating different range imaging cameras.

Error due to inharmonic properties of the signals: A periodic error can be observed depending on the nominal distance in the depth measurements due to the shape of the correlation function of the reference and received signal. This effect was first mentioned in [46] and is shown in figure 2.19. Experiments in [87] show that the error measured for different integration times taking into account the slight downwards slope has a range of about $50mm$ up from $2m$ distances. For closer distances the error introduced by near field effect (different *TOF* from the right and the left LED arrays) dominates over the error introduced by the inharmonic signals (see [77] for details).

Error due to pixel-wise offset: In [87] a constant pixel-wise offset in the depth measurement is reported. This is due to the different capacities of the pixels since being different physical parts. Therefore the signal is delayed by the own charge time of the capacitor of each of these parts. Since the capacity is constant over time, this offset will be as well constant, and will be visible in all measurements as a fixed pattern noise. Any technique for removing pattern noise in 2D cameras can be used to solve this problem.

Error due to amount of incident light: The amount of incident light effects the distance offset and depends on the nominal distance, the integration time and the reflectivity of the target. The non-linear dependency of the error on integration time and nominal distance can be observed in figure 2.19. This thesis mainly contributes to this topic. Impact estimations of this error source according to corresponding author is listed in table 2.3. Previous works such as [34], [46], [58] and [65] were studying this error. Studies of laser scanners which also determine the distance by means of Time of Flight also reported the effect of the target's reflectivity in the depth measurement [20, 59, 9].

Other error sources: There are some other sources of error which should be taken into account when using TOF Range Imaging Sensors. They are not considered in this work as they can be more or less controlled in an indoor environment, and/or have been previously studied by other authors.

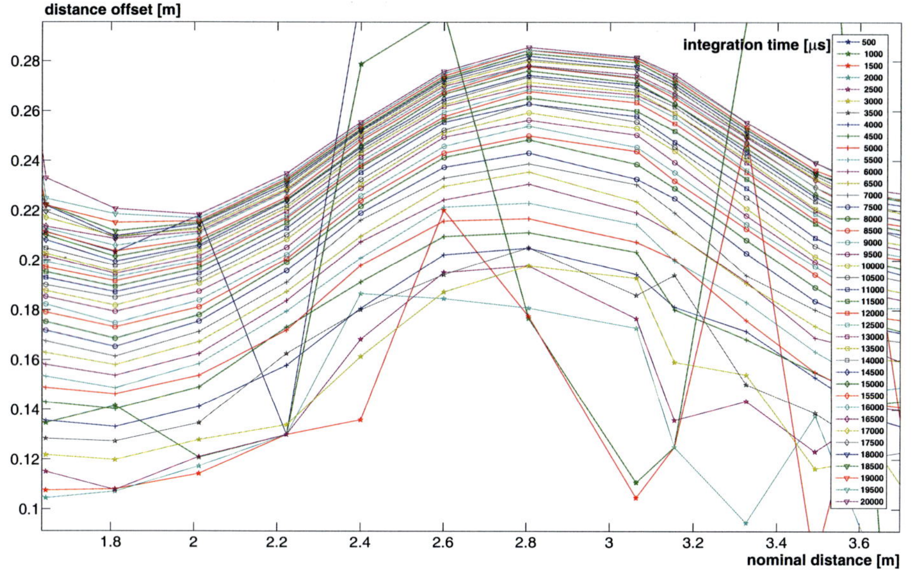

Figure 2.19: Distance error/offset $[m]$ plotted for different integration times in μs over the nominal distance $[m]$ for one target.

Errors due to additional IR source: Since the TOF range imaging sensor works on IR, obviously additional IR sources within the same bandwidth take effect on the distance measurement. Especially the high IR fraction of the sunlight disturbs the measurements as it reduces the amplitude by increasing the DC offset, as explained in [67] [65]. Some models of PMD Cameras incorporate a Suppression of Background Illumination (SBI) circuitry.

Errors due to temperature: The depth measurements drift with the camera's temperature, as reported in [46] or [65]. The warming up time of the camera is estimated to last about 15-20 min. The external temperature influencing for measurement precision has been estimated for the *CSEM SwissRanger SR-2* to be 8mm/°C [65].

Errors due to multi reflections: Reflections on the surrounding objects have an impact on the depth measurement. Measurements in this study were carried in an obstacle free environment. The work of Guðmundsson et al. does some basic investigation about this issue [34].

2.4.5 Research Activities in the Field of Depth Data Correction of TOF Range Imaging Cameras

Up to now many calibration methods for range imaging sensors have been proposed. Within this section the work related to the distance calibration is presented.

Although the work of Clark et al. [20] is not based on a range imaging sensor and rather on the *Leica HDS2500 laser scanner*, the work is briefly explained since the considered laser scanner also works on *IR-light* and focuses on the effects for the distance offset due to different target reflectivity´s. Within this work the average scanner measurement quality value against patch offset was measured. As reference for the average scanner measurement quality value *Neutral 8 Grey* was selected as the optimum in terms of reflectivity. Cubic regression curves were fitted to each set of data and were taken for distance correction. Since there appeared to be different regression curves for different bands of ranges, the correction factor was formulated only for a limited range (4 to 5.5m). As reason relating to this different discrete correction factors are assumed for different groups of ranges due to different manufacturers' calibration models.

May et al. [65] propose a calibration matrix in polar coordinates which is subtracted of the measurement data in order to correct the measured depth image that was captured with a *CSEM SwissRanger SR-2*. Within this lateral Look-up-table (LUT) calibration neither the *wiggling effect* nor the distance offset by the amount of incident light are corrected. As a reference a white wall is taken. There investigations focus on the automatic determination of an optimal integration time to avoid overexposure.

The method of Kuhnert [54] assumes a linear relation between phase and distance considering the 5x5 central pixels in combination with the standard deviation. For their investigations a *1k PMD-camera* with 64*x*16 pixel had been used. As factors that the proposed method is not able to master for distance correction the influence of target reflectivity for measurement precision and the nonlinear phase relation depending on the amplitude are indicated. It is assumed that the modulation image subsumes mentioned error sources. Therefore, to guarantee a certain measurement precision, the method is extended by a thresholding of 30% of the modulation ratio to identify distance measurements which cannot be corrected with the proposed calibration.

Investigating the *CSEM SwissRanger SR3000* Kahlmann et al. [46] first reported the so-called *wiggling effect* which characterizes the periodic behavior of the distance offset regarding the nominal distance and is shown in figure 2.19. The cause for the wiggling effect lies in the inharmonic properties of reference and incoming signal. Using a plane object with a homogenous reflectance property this behavior was determined for differ-

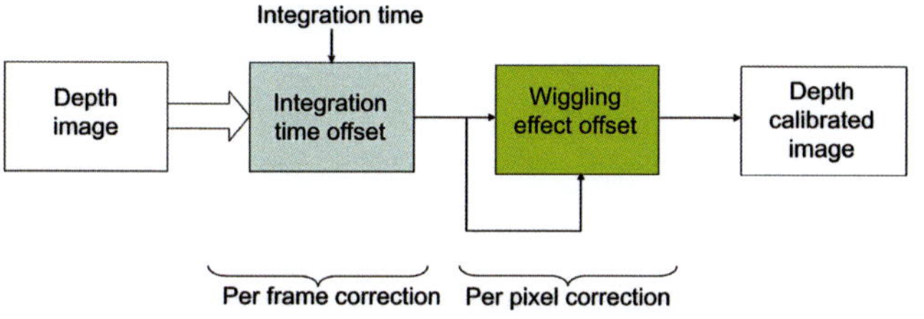

Figure 2.20: Look up table (LUT) based calibration method calibration method based on the investigations of Kahlmann et al. [46].

ent integration times and used as look-up tables for calibration. A linear interpolation is done for combinations of integration time and measured distance for which no LUT exists. In figure 2.20 the two-stage structure of the proposed calibration technique is shown. It calibrates out errors due to the pixel offset and the inharmonic behavior of the signals and partly calibrates out error depending on the amount of incident light by considering different integration times and nominal distances. The two-stage structure is as follows:

Stage 1 Calibrate integration times:
For one fixed distance to a target, acquire frames for the desired integration times. Take many frames for each integration time and average on time to reduce noise. Also correct the data by dropping overexposed pixels and calculating orthogonal depth, if not only central pixel are being considered. If it has not been automatically done, correct gate inhomogeneities and phase shift.

Stage 2 Calibrate pixel offset and inharmonic behavior:
For one fixed integration time, vary the distance to the target, moving over the whole range of distance wanted to measure. Acquire a frame (again with averaging over time and other corrections) for each distance. Correct the integration time offset by subtracting the vale resulting from stage 1. The acquired points should be used as a lookup table.

This calibration does not completely calibrate out the error due to the amount of incident light, since just considering different integration times and nominal distances. Therefore an error remains.

Lindner et al. [57] proposed a two stage calibration method based on investigations with the *PMD [vision] 3k* which handles the wiggling effect and corrects the central perspective. As target for reference distance capturing one planar, semireflective panel was used. The first stage of the calibration method reduces the distance offset for the whole image. The second stage pre-adapts per pixel for the first stage and postadapts the results of the

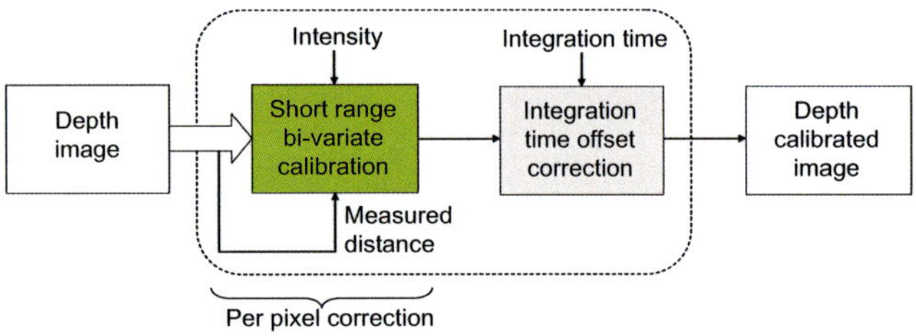

Figure 2.21: Structure of the depth calibration method proposed by Lindner et. al. [58].

global distance offset correction. The remaining distance error is less than $10mm$. Objects with different reflectance properties were not considered.

The work of Guðmundsson et al. [34] is based on the sensor *CSEM SwissRanger SR3000* and focuses on the external effects for the distance offset. Within their work they investigated the influence of the intensity on depth measurements. For the proposed calibration method they used the inversely proportional relation between distance offset and intensity. As it will be shown in section 4.1.4, this assumption is not valid for all distances. For evaluation reasons a plane object with regions with different reflectance properties at the distance of $\approx 0.81m$ had been used. For this certain setup the method showed a reduction of the offset to $10.9mm$.

Rapp [87] [86] analyzed three different range imaging sensors (*CSEM SwissRanger SR3000, PMD [vision] 19k and the Effektor O3D*). He proposed a calibration method for the whole distance range which handles the wiggling effect and the distance offset caused by the integration time. Objects with different reflectance properties are not handled by this method. The evaluation showed a maximum error span of $30mm$ considering a target with a homogeneous reflectivity for the *SR3000*.

Lindner et al. [58] used a *PMD [vision] 19k* for their investigations. The figure 2.21 shows the structure of the method proposed by them. They investigated the influence of different target reflectance properties by varying the integration time for a distance range between $0.9m$ and $1.9m$. They propose a two-stage method. The first is based on the assumption that systematic distance error and the error due to incident light are not independent. Therefore the distance error, e.g. wiggling effect, and the incident light error are handled together within the first stage. In figure 2.21 this stage is colored in dark green. The calibration model is extended by the integration time offset correction which is represented by the light grey box.

Gvili et. al. [35] used a *ZCam* for their investigations. Since they are the only research group that worked with the same camera the results are compared with their approach. They introduced a simple normalization stage to compensate for the different reflectivity coefficients. This is done be simply dividing the front portion pixel intensity $I_{front}(i,j)$ by the corresponding portion of the total intensity $I_{total}(i,j)$ yielding a corrected depth $D(i,j)$.

$$D(i,j) = \frac{I_{front}(i,j)}{I_{total}(i,j)} \tag{2.8}$$

This method does not consider any neighborhood and, hence, is a very fast method. But on the other side it neglects local information that should be incorporated for data correction to achieve a more stable data correction. Although this method yields sufficient data correction in case of near range and a small width of the light pulse, it fails when using the camera for a wide depth range like in our case with about $2m$ of range starting at $2m$ of distance so that we are considering a working range of $2-4m$.

3 Objectives of this work

The goal of this work is to develop a system that determines gait parameters of stroke patients for subsequent use in gait analysis and meets the demands for clinical every day use. The criteria for such a system are derived from the specific prerequisites for clinical every day use [14], [15]. They are grouped into *'Determination of relevant gait parameters'*, *'Accuracy'* and *'Clinical Applicability'*. They form the objectives of this work.

1st criterion *'Determination of relevant gait parameters'*:
In order to assess the gait characteristics of stroke patients, the following gait parameters need to be determined [41]. The most important parameter is the gait symmetry which is represented by the pelvis' movement trajectory. The reason for this is that stroke patients avoid the loading of the impaired leg. Also very important are the angles of the pelvis, hip, knee and ankle joint during the gait cycle. Their trajectories are considered for qualitative assessment by clinical professionals to evaluate a gait pattern. To look up, the gait characteristics of subjects after stroke are described in section 2.2.2.

2nd criterion *'Accuracy'*:
Generally, the gait parameters should be as accurate as possible. The determination of the accuracy is performed through a comparison of the determined gait parameters against reference gait parameters. Therefore, the limited accuracy of the reference gait parameters limits the accuracy that can be recognized. A markerbased system is used as measurement tool for acquiring the references because at the moment it is the most accurate measurement tool. It is described in detail in section 2.3.1.3. According to [56] the worst case mean squared error of such a system is $\epsilon = 7°$ for bone orientation which doubles for joint angles between two bones. The accuracy is closely related to the camera resolution which comprises the data accuracy and the spatial and temporal sample rate of the camera. The spatial resolution can be derived from ϵ. If assuming a limb length of $0.2m$ for the pelvis as the smallest limb, a minimum spatial resolution of $0.0130m$ is needed. Therefore, a depth resolution of $0.01m$ is set as requirement for the sensor. This resolution must be achieved for the volume in which the movement takes place.
A minimum required temporal sample rate of 15 Hz is considered to be sufficient for gait parameter determination [32], [41], because it is sufficient to detect gait pathology by the

therapist.
Another important factor is that the system must not influence the gait. That means that no measurement technology (e.g. markers or sensors) needs to be attached so that the gait pattern is not distorted [44], [60].

3rd criterion *'Clinical Applicability'*:
It relates to general applicability in clinical environment:

- A small system complexity increases the applicability. It refers to the number of cameras, their aiming and calibration as well to the system's dimensions which allows usage in normal-sized rooms.
- A small set-up time is an important factor because stroke patients suffer from quick exhaustion and clinical staff has a tight time table. According to [41] a set-up time of less than 5 minutes is required for stroke patients.
- A high processing rate enables the system for therapy simultaneous gait parameter determination. However, this is no mandatory criterion because post processing is sufficient at first.
- The clinical acceptance of the provided gait parameters. This means that the gait parameters need to be presented in a form that corresponds to accepted clinical concepts. Figure 3.1 shows gait parameter trajectories which were generated with a commercial markerbased system and how it is commonly used for gait analysis by clinical staff.

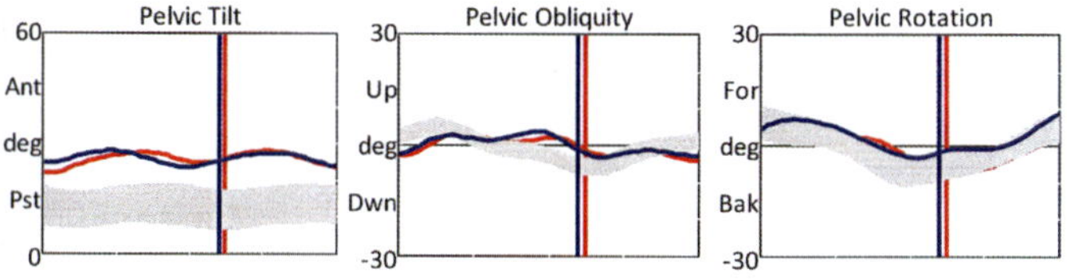

Figure 3.1: Example of the representation of gait parameter data. The gray region represents the reference range and the blue and red graph the trajectory of the left and right joint angles. Extracted from [88].

For this work the applicability for the *HapticWalker* forms a special requirement. In table 3.1 on page 40 the different approaches and research activities for gait parameter capturing, which were presented in section 2.3, are assessed through the above criteria. It shows that neither of the presented research activities provide a non-complex system architecture and accurate measurement of the relevant gait characteristics while coping with the prerequisites of the targeted demonstration scenario.

		BioMotion, Stanford University	*IESK, Universität Magdeburg*	*IMM, TU of Denmark*	*Dept. Biomed. Eng., Kyung Hee University, South Korea*	*ECS, University of Southampton*
Capture relevant gait characteristics		✓	✓	✗, no pelvis modeled, only cadence and step length, sagittal joint angles	✗, not specified	✗, no pelvis modeled, only sagittal movements
measurement accuracy	sensor resolution	resolution depends on number and poses of cameras and movements, ≈ 15% volumetric error for 8 ideally placed cameras [68]. 200 *Hz*	depth only for predefined planes, must be aligned with object movement 20 *Hz*	±20 mm depth image 54 *Hz*, 176 × 144pxl	theoretical depth resolution of ≈ 12cm at 2.5m distance. Additional systematic error for concave objects, 48 *Hz* 640×480	no depth, 5-30 *Hz*, 170 × 128-1024 × 768 pxl
	gait parameter accuracy	accurate*	position accurate, joint angles moderate* (apply movement pattern model), no accurate pelvis joint angles	okay* (apply movement pattern model), no internal rotation, no hip modeling, only cadence and step length, sagittal joint angles	moderate*	okay* only sagittal movements, no internal rotation
Clinical Applicability	small system dimensions	min. 8 2D-cameras, cameras circularly placed around object ⇒ $12m \times 12m$ space requirement*	8 2D-cameras, ⇒ $4m \times 4m$ space requirement*	1 2.5D-camera, ⇒ $2m \times 3.5m$ space requirement*	1 stereo camera system, ⇒ $3m \times 7m$ space requirement*	1 2D-camera, ⇒ $2m \times 5m$ space requirement*
	set-up time	-, but model parameterization, model init	-, but movement model learning, model parameterization and init	-, but movement model learning	-, but model init	-, but model parameterization, model init
	processing rate	3:00 h for 400 images*	-	-	-	-
	clinical acceptance	✓	✓	✗	✗	✗
	applicability at demonstration scenario	✗, bars and patient suspension obstruct camera view	✓	✗, model implies movement pattern that deranges gait parameters.	✓	✗, just 2D data, sagittal movements

Table 3.1: This table provides an overview of the research activities for marker free optical systems for gait parameter determination. The asterisk (*) marks values that are not explicitly given but estimated. (✓≡ 'yes', ✗≡ 'no'), (-≡ not specified)

Within this work a system for gait parameter determination of stroke patients shall be realized that meets the above mentioned criteria and thereby outlines existing work. The system is realized markerless to ensure that the realized system does not alter the movements of the patient because no markers are attached. This also ensures that small set-up time is needed.

Another outline is formed by the use of a TOF camera, because up to now no other research group uses a TOF camera for gait parameter determination. There is a system that applies a TOF camera [43], but it only uses the depth information for segmentation purpose from a side view on the patient and not for direct determination of the gait parameters. Therefore, the presented work outlines existing work by considering a frontal view and directly incorporating the depth information into the gait parameter determination.

The single-view TOF camera results in a low system complexity while providing depth information. Since it is just one camera, it is non-spacious and non-complex. Additionally, it is suited for use at the *HapticWalker* because it copes with the bars and the weight suspension. This overcomes complex multi-camera systems that use *SfS* such as the work from Stanford [19] which are spacious and need an unobstructed view for all cameras and, therefore, cannot cope with the bars and the weight suspension of the *HapticWalker*. The drawback of the multi-camera system such as [17] is the complex adjustment of the camera set-up according to the captured movements and the need of the patient to walk along that specific trail. Standard single-view 2D camera systems overcome the disadvantages of complex multi-camera systems, but lack depth information. Therefore, these approaches yield limited information for out-of-projection-plane movements which requires sophisticated models to overcome this drawback on high computational costs.

Therefore, by using the TOF camera, a new promising path is taken and the developed system serves as a contribution to the applicability of TOF range imaging cameras for human motion analysis. Due to the novelty of the camera technology, the camera shows systematic errors that have not been fully investigated and compensated up to now. Therefore, one major objective of this work is to compensate these shortcomings and improve the accuracy of the depth data so that it meets the criterion of a minimum resolution of 0.01m.

The demonstrator *HapticWalker* defines the working space that must be covered by the realized system. The work space is defined by a body height of 1.91m (*DIN 33402* [74]), which refers to the height of the 95-percentile of men in Germany, and the range of movements of the captured person. The range of the horizontal movements is given by the *HapticWalker* with 1.10m. Because of the chosen sensor view a distance range between 2.0m and 3.5m needs to be covered.

Although this work focuses on the extraction of gait parameters for gait analysis, the applicability of the system concerning the determination of other movements and within other operation fields is always kept in mind. This is an additional important share of the developed solution for future work such as for *man-robot-cooperation* in industrial applications, e. g., to continue the research works [51],[53]. Additionally, the single view TOF range imaging camera forms an excellent platform for *home rehabilitation* for future work due to its easy set-up and its little space requirement.

4 Concept for Gait Parameter Determination

This chapter deals with the concept of the realized system for gait parameter determination. Figure 4.1 shows an overview of the realized system for two subsequent frames (time step t and t-1). The blue boxes represent processes, while the white boxes represent result data that is passed allong the arrows to the next process. Every time step the Time-of-Flight (TOF) camera captures a depth image which is then passed to the depth data correction stage which is marked with ① in the figure. With the corrected $2\frac{1}{2}$D data and initialized through the results of the previous frame a 3D body model is fitted into the data so that the posture of the body model corresponds to the posture of the captured human ②. The general idea of fitting a 3D-model in 3D-data forms an already known

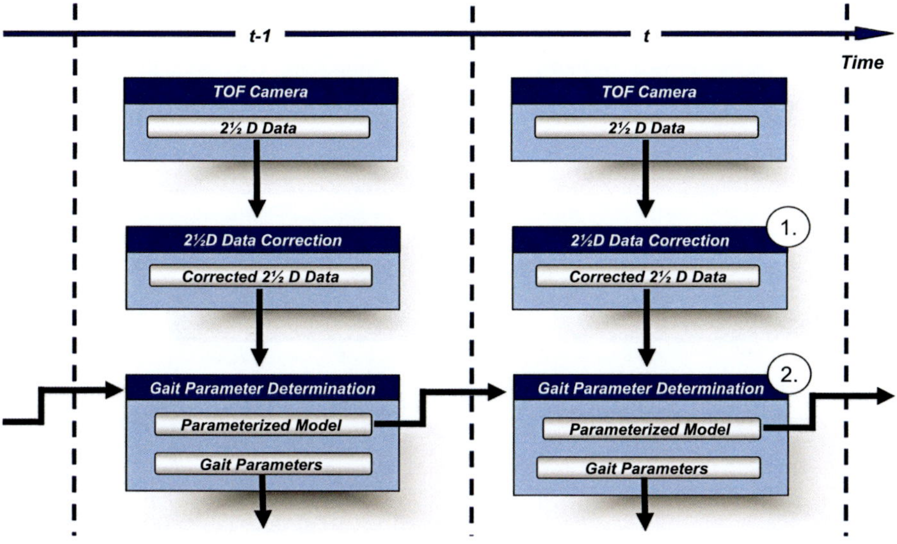

Figure 4.1: Overview of the processing pipeline from the TOF camera to the gait parameters of the realized system for two subsequent frames (time step t and t-1). It illustrates the interaction of the two main components of this work.

approach which performance early had been proven by [27]. The gait parameter are then determined of the poses of the body model segments, i. e., the joint angles are retrieved from the poses of two physiologically connected body segments. An example for this is the knee angle which is defined by the pose of the thigh and the shank.

The sensory base of the system is a TOF depth camera because it meets the demands for an easy integration due to a lower complexity compared with a multi camera system as discussed in section 3. But TOF cameras are not directly applicable for the determination of gait parameter because their data show a relatively high degree of noise and inherent systematic errors which exceed the accuracy requirements of the considered application. Up to now these errors are not handled sufficiently (see section 2.4.4). Therefore, an important part of this work deals with the data correction of the TOF camera data which is described in section 4.1. After the correction of the data, the posture of the captured human is synthesized by the body model fitting and the gait parameters are extracted from the body model. This is described in section 4.2.

4.1 Concept for Depth Data Correction of TOF Cameras

TOF cameras are a relatively new type of sensor. Therefore, many problems such as the low resolution of the depth data have not been solved yet. For this reason TOF cameras cannot be directly applied for gait parameter determination. Therefore, this section ad-

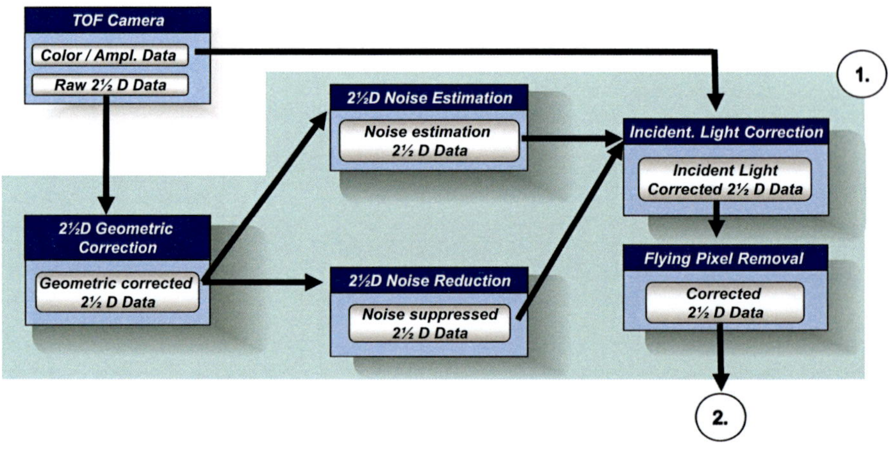

Figure 4.2: Overview of the depth data correction pipeline which passes the corrected $2\frac{1}{2}$D data as output to the *'gait parameter determination'* stage. It corresponds to ① in figure 4.1

dresses the depth data enhancement to achieve the applicability of TOF cameras for gait parameter determination.

The depth data enhancement consists of four different stages each of which addresses a different error source. The components of the depth data enhancement are *geometric correction, noise reduction, incident light correction* and *Flying Pixel Removal*. The concept with the components for the data enhancement is illustrated in figure 4.2. A section is devoted to each component.

In this thesis, two TOF camera models were investigated, the *PMD [vision] 19k* and the *3DVSystems ZCam*. For the depth data enhancement for both cameras the same conceptual strategy was followed. The implementation of the components differs for the incident light correction due to their different characteristics while being equal for the remaining components. This is due to the different features the cameras offer such as the color channel for the *ZCam* or the raw data sample data of the *PMD [vision] 19k*. Before the components of the data enhancement are presented the used camera projection model is described. This is important for the geometric projection correction and the reconstruction of the 3D data out of the $2\frac{1}{2}$D data.

Figure 4.3 gives an impression of the quality of the raw depth data (a) and of the depth data enhancement results (b).

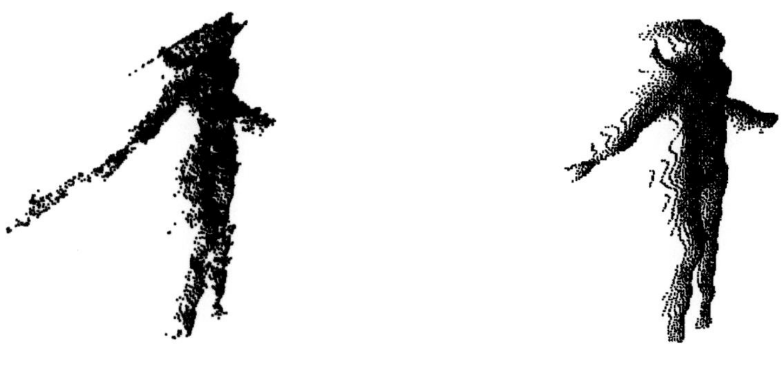

(a) (b)

Figure 4.3: Foreground segmented depth data of the same frame viewed from the same perspective, (a) without any error correction and (b) with proposed $2\frac{1}{2}$D data error correction.

4.1.1 Camera Projection Model for 3D Reconstruction

This section describes the camera projection model for a $2\frac{1}{2}$D camera and how it is used in this work with respect to the standardly used 2D camera model.
The TOF range imaging camera uses a standard lens and camera geometry and, therefore, resembles the pinhole camera. With this assumption the projection of a point $\vec{X} = (X,Y,Z)^T \in \mathbb{R}^3$ onto a point $\vec{x} = (x,y)^T \in \mathbb{R}^2$ on the sensor plane can be characterized by the camera projection matrix, according to [11]:

$$\mathbf{P} = \underbrace{\begin{bmatrix} f_x & \alpha_c \cdot f_x & p_x \\ 0 & f_y & p_y \\ 0 & 0 & 1 \end{bmatrix}}_{\mathbf{K}} \cdot \mathbf{R} \cdot [\mathbf{I} - \widetilde{\mathbf{C}}] \tag{4.1}$$

The matrix $\mathbf{K}$ is the camera calibration matrix, $\mathbf{R}$ is the rotation matrix and $\mathbf{I}$ is a 3×3 identity matrix. $\widetilde{\mathbf{C}}$ is the origin of the camera given in 3D world coordinates. The coefficients of $\mathbf{K}$ are the foci f_x and f_y along the x- and y-axis, the central projection point $\vec{p_{cp}}(p_x, p_y)$ on the sensor plane and the skew coefficient α_c. The skew coefficient represents the angle between the pixel axes $\vec{a_x}$ and $\vec{a_y}$, which is normally assumed to be 90° after [36]:

$$\alpha_c = \angle(\vec{a_x}, \vec{a_y}) - \frac{\pi}{2}[rad] \tag{4.2}$$

A projection of $\vec{X} = (X,Y,Z)^T$ onto a point $\vec{x} = (x,y)^T$ is defined by:

$$\vec{x} = \mathbf{P} \cdot \vec{X} \tag{4.3}$$

Here, the third dimension of $\vec{X}$ is lost.
In case of using a TOF range imaging camera instead, the third dimension of $\vec{X}$ is represented by a scalar, the depth $d(\vec{x})$. The homogeneous 3D point $\vec{X}$ is therefore projected to the homogeneous $2\frac{1}{2}$D point $\vec{x}$ according to:

$$d(\vec{x})\vec{x} = \mathbf{P} \cdot \vec{X} \tag{4.4}$$

For the opposite direction of the projection, this means that a 3D point $\vec{X}$ can be reconstructed unambiguously on the base of a $2\frac{1}{2}$D point $\vec{x}$ through the scaling depth $d(\vec{x})$:

$$\vec{X} = d(\vec{x})\mathbf{R}\mathbf{K}^{-1}\vec{x} + \widetilde{\mathbf{C}} \tag{4.5}$$

This equation is used for the reconstruction of the 3D points $\vec{X}$ on the base of the $2\frac{1}{2}$D points $\vec{x}$ which are captured with the TOF camera.
Because the camera center is chosen as the world coordinate center, $\widetilde{\mathbf{C}}$ vanishes. The stationary camera position allows the world coordinate system to be aligned according to the camera so that the rotation matrix $\mathbf{R}$ becomes the identity matrix $\mathbf{I}$.

4.1.2 Depth Data Enhancement by Geometric Projection Correction

As shown in figure 4.2, the 'Geometric Projection Correction' is the first stage of the data correction processing pipeline.

Projection errors which result from imperfect lenses are standardly compensated by camera lens calibration. But the lens calibration effects the projection onto the sensor plane only and not the length of the optical path which is the base for the depth measure of TOF cameras. Therefore, the current lens calibration approaches are not comprehensive enough to handle TOF depth cameras. Therefore, the standard lens calibration just forms one part of the correction of the TOF camera. The correction of the optical path length has not been investigated up to now by any other research group. This section focuses on the lens correction of the TOF depth camera including the optical path length. Before depth data correction, the correction for 2D cameras is described.

There are two approaches for 2D lens distortion correction; *model based* and the *mapping based* approach. The *model-based* approach uses models of the lens whose parameters are determined in the calibration process. This approach is possible when conventional lenses are used and there are lens calibration models for these lenses. The *mapping-based* approach basically uses a Look-Up-Table (LUT) which is built from sample data. It is applied when non-conventional lenses are used.
The considered TOF cameras both use conventional lenses. Therefore, a *model-based* calibration approach is applied. The resulting intrinsic camera parameters define the camera calibration matrix **K** (see eq. 4.1). For the identification of the intrinsic camera parameters the method from [11] is applied. As valid simplification the skew coefficient α_c is assumed to be zero [36]. Additionally, the coefficients of radial and tangential lens distortion $k_1, \ldots, k_5$ are determined. These coefficients parameterize a polynomial approximation of the lens distortion which forms the calibration model.
The undistorted 2D image point $\vec{x} = (x, y)^T$ is computed from the distorted 2D image point $\vec{x}_d = (x_d, y_d)^T$ by first correcting the lens distortion to get a normalized undistorted image point and then multiplying the camera matrix. For this first the above mentioned coefficients are determined with the help of a normalized pinhole projection $\vec{\tilde{x}} = (\tilde{x}, \tilde{y})^T = (\tilde{X}/\tilde{Z}, \tilde{Y}/\tilde{Z})^T$ of a know points $\vec{\tilde{X}} = (\tilde{X}, \tilde{Y}, \tilde{Z})^T$ in 3D space. These are given by checkerboards and their known structure. Sample images of the checkerboard are displayed in figure 4.4.

The new coordinate of the normalized undistorted point $\vec{\tilde{x}}_d = (\tilde{x}_d, \tilde{y}_d)$ is computed by summing up the radial and the tangential undistortion:

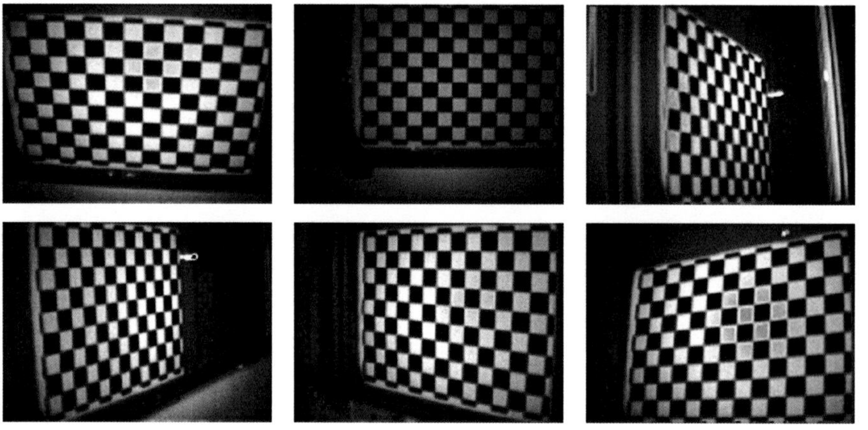

Figure 4.4: Calibration checkerboards from different views used for intrinsic parameter determination.

The radial undistorted 2D image coordinates x_r and y_r are computed through with $r^2 = \widetilde{x}^2 + \widetilde{y}^2$:

$$\begin{pmatrix} x_r \\ y_r \end{pmatrix} = (1 + k_1 \cdot r^2 + k_2 \cdot r^4 + k_5 \cdot r^6) \begin{pmatrix} \widetilde{x} \\ \widetilde{y} \end{pmatrix} \tag{4.6}$$

The tangential undistorted 2D image coordinates x_t and y_t are computed by:

$$\begin{pmatrix} x_t \\ y_t \end{pmatrix} = \begin{pmatrix} 2 \cdot k_3 \cdot \widetilde{x} \cdot \widetilde{y} + k_4(\widetilde{x}^2 + \widetilde{y}^2)^2 + 2 \cdot \widetilde{x}^2 \\ k_3 \cdot (r^2 + 2 \cdot \widetilde{y}^2) + 2 \cdot k_4 \cdot \widetilde{x} \cdot \widetilde{y} \end{pmatrix} \tag{4.7}$$

The reader is referred for information about the derivation of the polynomials to [11].

The *model-based* approach is designed for 2D cameras, but not for TOF range image cameras. Therefore, it just compensates for the 2D lens distortions. This is not sufficient for TOF cameras.

In contrast to the 2D cameras not only the erroneous projection point on the sensor plane needs to be corrected but also the optical path length because this is the source for the Time-of-Flight measurement. This interrelationship is schematically illustrated in figure 4.5. The orange line represents the optical path of camera. The blue area represents the band of possible optical paths limited by the lens aperture. The dark blue line is the mean optical path of this band. When comparing the two paths the absolute values of the covered distance differ. This is not critical for 3D to 2D projection but affects the measured depth data. When we try to reconstruct a homogeneous 3D point $\vec{X}$ of the projected $2\frac{1}{2}$D point $d(\vec{x})\vec{x}$ an erroneous 3D point $\vec{X}_d$ with a distance error d_d in all three dimensions $(X, Y, Z)^T$ result.

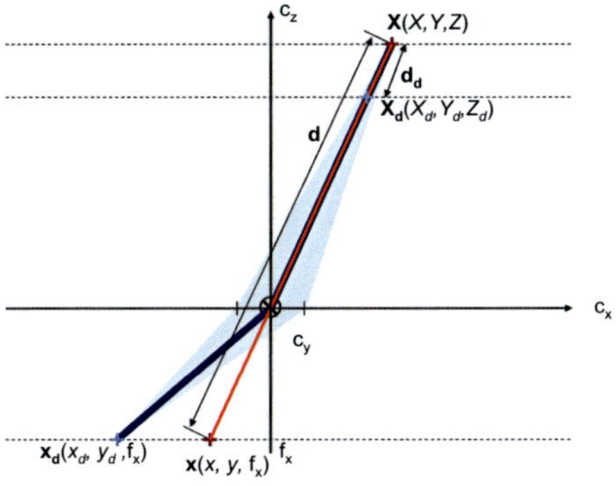

Figure 4.5: Depth measurement error introduced by the lens distortion. The orange line represents the optical path of the camera. The blue area represents the band of possible optical paths limited by the lens aperture, the dark blue line is the mean optical path. A comparison of the two lines differs in the absolute values of the covered distance which affect the depth measurement.

To analyze the distance error d_d, the difference between the lengths of the optical paths is determined. Because the differences of the paths occurs inside the camera, the error d_d can be determined through some vector analysis. See figure 4.5 for visualization. Here, the distance error d_d results from two vectors. These are: the vector of the distorted 3D point $\vec{X_d}$ and of the undistorted $\vec{X}$ with $\vec{S} = (0, 0, -f_x)^T$ and $M_{3\times2} = [1\,0; 0\,1; 0\,0]$.

$$\vec{X_d} = M_{3\times2} \cdot \vec{x_d} + \vec{S} = (x_d, y_d, -f_x)^T \qquad (4.8)$$
$$\vec{X} = M_{3\times2} \cdot \vec{x} + \vec{S} = (x, y, -f_x)^T$$

The distance error d_d can be calculated by subtracting the absolute values of these vectors:

$$d_d = \|\vec{X_d}\| - \|\vec{X}\| = \sqrt{\|x_d^2 - x^2\| + \|y_d^2 - y^2\|} \qquad (4.9)$$

When taking a lateral deviation of only a few pixels and the dimensions of the pixels of the camera into account it appears obvious that the distance error d_d on the depth measurement is small and, therefore, can be neglected. Even with a maximum lateral lens distortion of half the sensor size, d_d would sum up to less than $\approx 2mm$ with a standard lens with a focus $f = 12mm$ and an opening angle of 40° which is given for the *PMD [vision] 19k*. If capturing an object at $2.5m$ distance, the distance error d_d would amount to $\leq 1‰$ of the optical path.

Therefore, at the moment with the current performance of the TOF range imaging cameras the depth measurement error induced by the geometric distortion is insignificant.

As we shall see in the next section, there are currently more important error sources to investigate and compensate.

4.1.3 Depth Data Enhancement by Noise Reduction

Depth data captured with a TOF camera comprise a relatively high noise level. This is apparent by the mere look at the depth data image in figure 4.6(a).
Due to its nonlinear characteristics, noise normally is suppressed with a non linear filter, such as the *median filter*. Because of the noise strength, the necessary window size to reduce the noise needed to be ≥ 9. Applying a filter with such a big window size affects important structures, i. e., between the legs at the crotch. At these regions the application of a median filter results in displaced object borders.
Therefore, another approach is chosen. Opening-closing / closing-opening filters are applied to suppress the noise that appears as dark and light structures of different size. Thereby, closing removes dark structures and opening the light ones. In the case of interference with both large and small structures as in our case simply applying opening-closing / closing-opening filters with a large structural element do not lead to the desired results.
Therefore, it was chosen to create an *alternating sequential filtering* (ASF) in combination with a toggle criterion which is called *toggle mapping* and is described in [95], [97]. The alternating sequential filtering works as follows.

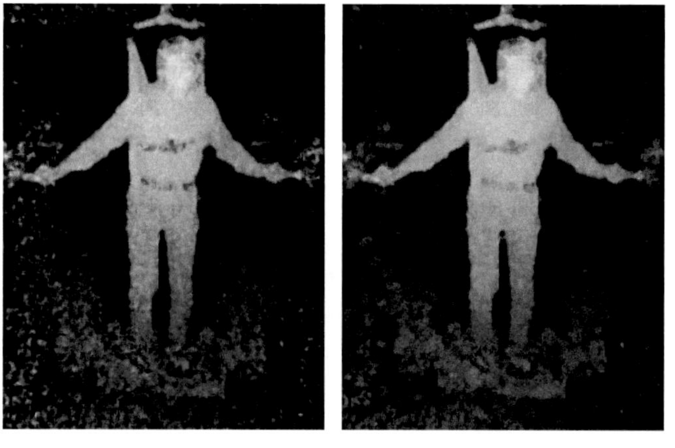

(a) (b)

Figure 4.6: (a) Input depth data d and (b) the output depth data d_{corr}^{NR} of the noise reduction stage.

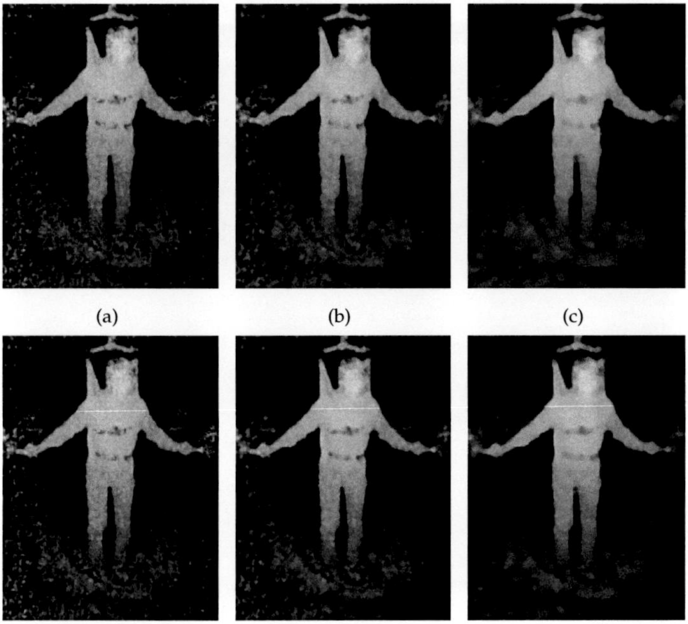

(a) (b) (c) (d) (e) (f)

Figure 4.7: Intermediate results of the noise reduction by *ASF*. (a) is the first intermediate result M_1, (b) the second (M_3) and (c) the third (M_5). According to this, (d) displays N_1, (e) is N_3 and (f) shows N_5.

Let γ_i be the *opening* and ϕ_i its counterpart *closing* of size i. The considered dual morphological filters 'opening-closing' and 'closing-opening' are:

$$
\begin{aligned}
m_i =& \gamma_i\left[\phi_i(d)\right] = \gamma_i\phi_i \\
n_i =& \phi_i\left[\gamma_i(d)\right] = \phi_i\gamma_i
\end{aligned}
\tag{4.10}
$$

With this an ASF of size i is defined by the sequential application of the filters m_i and n_i, starting with the size 1 up to the size i.:

$$
\begin{aligned}
M_i =& m_i \dots m_2 m_1 \\
N_i =& n_i \dots n_2 n_1
\end{aligned}
\tag{4.11}
$$

The *toggle mapping* is a two stage method. The ASF forms the first stage and defines the elements of the transformation so that the family of transformations ψ is $\{M_i, N_i, \dots, M_1, N_1, I\}$ with I being the identity transformation. The second stage is a decision rule stage (the *toggle criterion*) in which a value is selected from the ASF results. The selection is performed with the so-called morphological center β. These processing stages to compute the noise reduced depth data d_{corr}^{NR} can be written as:

$$d_{corr}^{NR} = \beta = (I \vee \underbrace{\bigwedge_i \psi_i}_{\substack{\text{pointwise}\\ \text{minimum}}}) \wedge \underbrace{\bigvee_i \psi_i}_{\substack{\text{pointwise}\\ \text{maximum}}} \tag{4.12}$$

In the simple case of $i = 2$ this equation simplifies to a median filtering. The intermediate results of this procedure are shown in figure 4.7. Here, the images show three iterations of M_i and N_i for $i = \{1, 3, 5\}$. The result of the noise reduction is shown in figure 4.6(b).

4.1.4 Depth Data Enhancement by Incident Light Correction

This section refers to the correction of the depth data with respect to the incident light, i. e., the amount of light that is reflected by the captured objects.
Within this section the investigations concerning the incident light are described for the two considered TOF cameras; first for the *PMD [vision] 19k* (see section 4.1.4.1) then for the *ZCam* (see section 4.1.4.2).
Due to the novelty of TOF cameras and the lack of comprehensive studies, an intensive study of the depth data generated by these cameras preceded the development of a depth data enhancement. The data acquisition for this study is principally the same for both investigated depth cameras. Because of some differences, the study will be explained more in detail for the *PMD [vision] 19k*, which comes first, than for the *ZCam* where just specifics are presented that differ from the other data acquisition process.

4.1.4.1 Incident Light Correction for the *PMD [vision] 19k*

The raw depth data has a set of systematic distance errors which depend on the distance to the object, the integration time and the amount of incident light, whereas the latter parameter depends on the first two. Additionally, the amount of incident light also depends on the reflectivity and the orientation of the object. For the *PMD [vision] 19k* the amount of incident light is represented by the data amplitude *Ampl* (see section 2.4.3.1).

To investigate the relations between these parameters and their influences on the distance measure, the distance error is investigated separately for these parameters. Here, the distance error is defined as the measured distance minus the nominal distance.
The influence of different reflectance properties is approached by investigating different targets with different reflectivities. The targets are of nearly Lambertian reflectance to reduce the effect of orientation on the investigations. Additionally, all targets are positioned orthogonally to the depth camera to provide a constant measurement environment. The orthogonality is achieved by a setup shown in figure 4.8 that is based on two laser range

finders. These laser range finders are attached on both sides of the depth camera with a constant base distance ($b = 350mm$). The mean of both laser range finders that feature an accuracy of $\pm 2mm$ was used for nominal distances measurement. The laser range finders emit a laser to point at a mark on the wall the targets are attached to. These marks have the same base distance b as the laser range finders sideways of the depth camera so that a precise alignment can be achieved. Regardless of the nominal distance this setup results in a maximum angle error $\alpha = arctan(rfe_{max}/b) \approx 0.7°$ for the maximum accumulated distance error of the two laser range finders $rfe_{max} = 4mm$.

The considered nominal distance ranges from $2m$ to $7m$ with a $0.5m$ step width. A variety of targets with different reflectance properties and integration times between $6ms$ and $60ms$ were applied in this data evaluation study. For the data evaluation it is assumed that when keeping nominal distance and integration time constant the differences between errors of different targets are due to their different reflectance properties.

All the measurements have been made after a warming up period of the camera of 30 minutes like proposed by Kahlmann et. al. in [46]. Additionally, all measurements have been denoised by temporal and spatial averaging. The averaging strategy was a 5×5 spatial median because of the small sample size and averaging over 10 frames. This technique had shown a good performance in preliminary studies related with the wiggling effect error (see figure 2.19 at page 33).
In contrast to the *3DVSystems ZCam*, one characteristic of the *PMD [vision] 19k* is that the camera is not normalizing the data so that over- and underexposure occur. Therefore, the

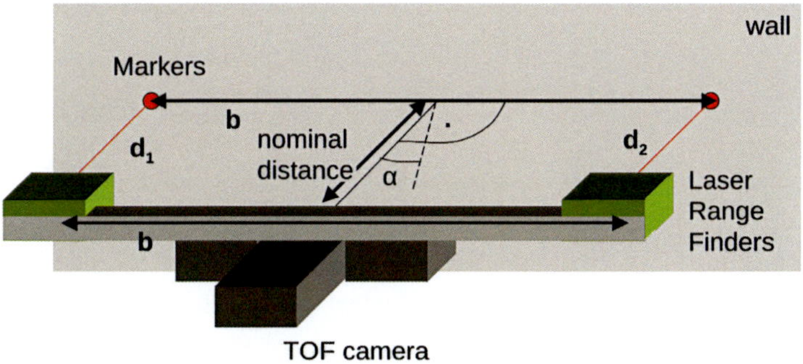

Figure 4.8: Measurement setup for the determination of the distance error of the TOF camera. The range finders are placed at the ends of the camera construction and aimed towards the wall in parallel with the camera in direction α. This is achieved by aiming the laser range finders on two marks on the wall which are at the same height as the camera.

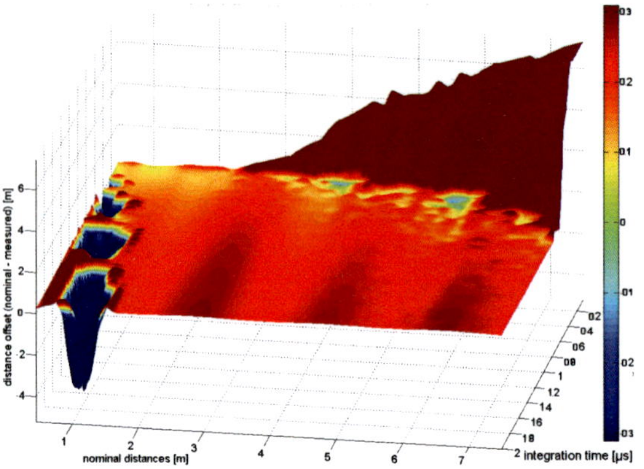

Figure 4.9: Distance error to nominal distance for integration times between 0.2 and 20 ms for a target with a homogeneous reflectivity. Over- and underexposed distance measurements as well as the wiggling effect is present.

appearance of under- and overexposed pixel needs to be identified and processed in a robust way.

In figure 4.9 the distance error over integration time [μs] and nominal distance [m] for one target is shown. Overexposed pixels can clearly be identified on the left side (*'the hole'*) where a target at little nominal distance is captured with a long integration time. Underexposed pixels appear for a big nominal distance and a short integration time (the dark red elevation at the backmost part of the plot).

In the figure 4.10 the data amplitude *Ampl* that represent the amount of the incident light see section 2.4.3.1) is shown over nominal distance and integration time. It can be noted that underexposed pixels can be robustly identified by simply thresholding the amplitude. For overexposed pixels the amplitude falls off when the received light exceeds a certain value. This fact that shows up with raw values exceeding a certain value is exploited for the identification of overexposed pixels as published in [85]. Like overexposed pixels the underexposed pixels are discarded when the *Ampl* of the considered pixel falls below a certain value.

To increase the distance range in which the camera data is not over- or underexposed, the integration time is toggled. This means that at least two images are captured with different integration times and combining the data. This widely spread approach of toggling the integration time is not followed because this would reduce the frame rate to less than 7 *Hz* which is not enough for the considered application of gait parameter determination (see section 3).

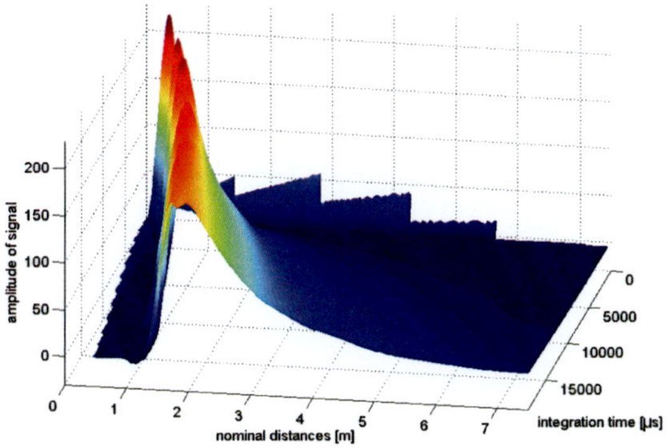

Figure 4.10: Corresponding amplitude to nominal distance for integration times between 0.2 and 20 ms.

To reiterate, for the investigation nominal distances between $2m$ and $7m$ are considered with a step width of $0.5m$. At these nominal distances the distances are measured with TOF camera for a variety of targets of different reflectance property at and integration times between $6ms$ and $60ms$. These measurements show that different reflectance properties affect the distance error depending on the nominal distances and the integration time in a different way.

The behavior is shown in figure 4.11 and has first been published through this research group [79]. In the figure each plot represents a single nominal distance (2m, 3m, 4m, 5m, 6m and 7m). The upper figures 4.11(a) and (b) that represent the nominal distance of $2m$ and of $3m$ show an increase of the distance error with the amplitude. This behavior inverts with bigger nominal distances, as shown in the four lower figures (c), (d), (e) and (f). Here, the offset decreases inversely proportional with the amplitude. Additionally, it can be noticed that the distance error varies with the integration time. Because this

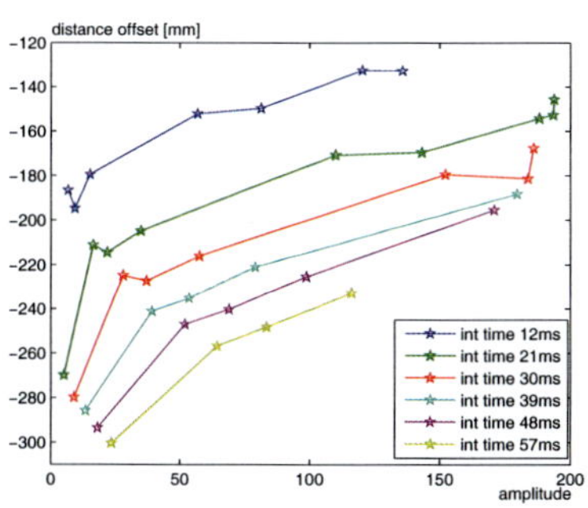

(a)

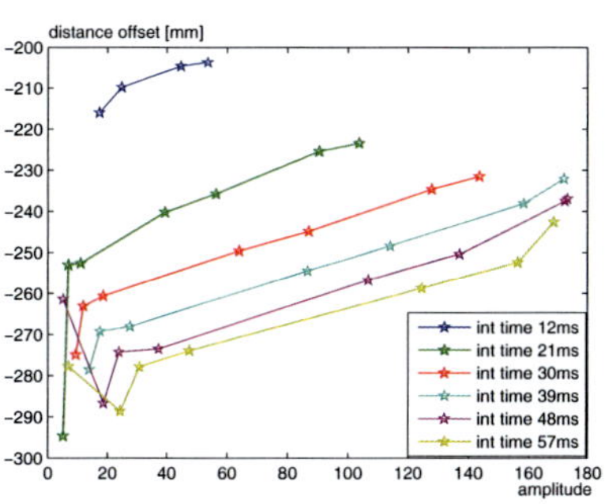

(b)

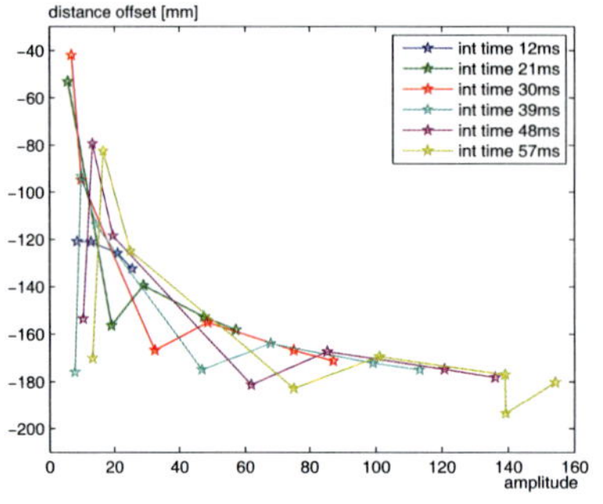

(c)

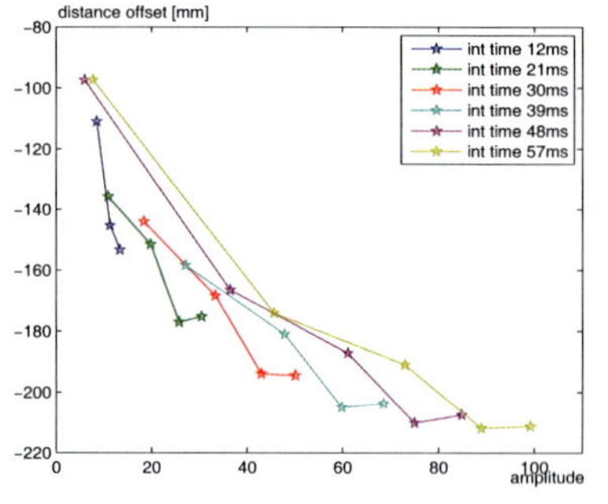

(d)

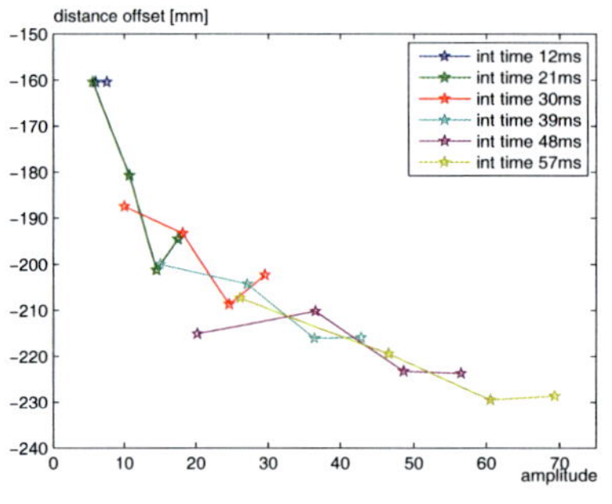

(e)

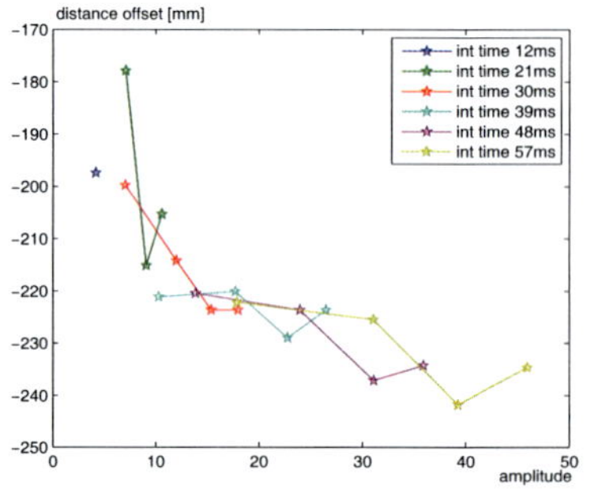

(f)

Figure 4.11: The distance errors (offsets) for different integration times against the amplitude values. Each of the plots refer to a different nominal distance (2*m* (a), 3*m* (b), 4*m* (c), 5*m* (d), 6*m* (e), and 7*m* (f)). (a) and (b) show an increase over the amplitude and (c), (d), (e), and (f) show a decrease over the amplitude.

distance error is not constant regarding the distance, it can not be handled with the LUT's proposed by [46].
A method is proposed which exploits this effect for depth data correction.

The proposed method distinguishes the parts of the distance and integration time related errors which are independent on the incident light and those which are dependent.
The structure of the method is shown in figure 4.12. There it can be seen that the proposed calibration method consists of three stages. The first two handle integration time and wiggling effect offsets in the same way as proposed in [46], [57], [87]. They correspond to the incident light-independent part of the integration time and distance errors, respectively, and have to be done first because reliable data is needed for the third stage.

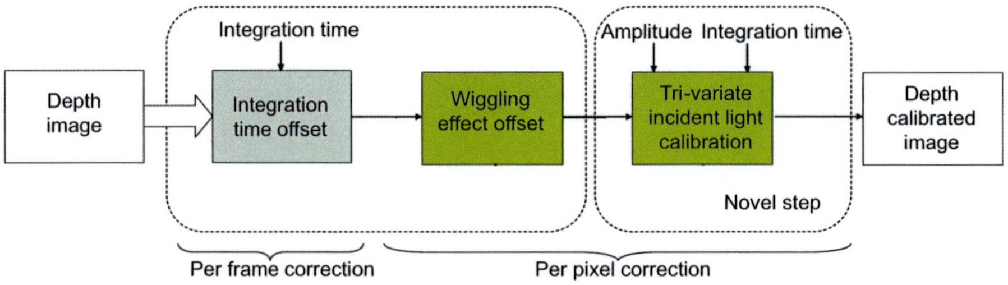

Figure 4.12: The structure of the proposed calibration method.

The third and novel stage incorporates the error due to the variation of the incident light in a novel way, combining the amplitude, the integration time and the measured distance.

1. The first stage in figure 4.12 is a LUT-based correction which calibrates out the integration time offset. The LUT is constructed by measuring the distances for a fixed nominal distance, a fixed target and an interest range of integration times (between 6 and 60*ms*). The wiggling effect offset is subtracted and it is assumed that the distance errors, which remain between different integration times, are due to the integration time.
2. The second stage handles the wiggling effect for which another LUT is constructed. Taking a white target and an integration time of 20*ms* as reference, 50 samples between 2*m* and 6*m* were taken. With these samples a *B-Spline* fitting for the LUT's is applied.
3. The plots in the figure 4.14 show that the dependence of distance error from the amplitude varies with the distances and the integration time in a non-trivial way. Therefore, it is not possible to use only one LUT to handle the incident light-related distance error for all distances and integration time ranges. The third stage, therefore, incorporates the incident light effect for calibration in a tri-variate approach as a novelty. A set of LUT's is used, one for every desired nominal distance and integration time. The proposed calibration method uses amplitude, integration time and up to then-corrected distance data at the same time for correction. In order to know which distance-integration time LUT has to be applied, the 'up to the point' corrected distance is used. With a precision of 50*mm* this data is precise enough to determine the proper LUT for the final correction of the distance.

For the above study of the depth data it is sufficient to consider the central pixels only. To correct the whole depth image, it is necessary to deal with the pixel-wise distance error which is dependent on the location in the depth image. Because this depth error origins in the non-uniform illumination of the scene by the TOF camera, an illumination model

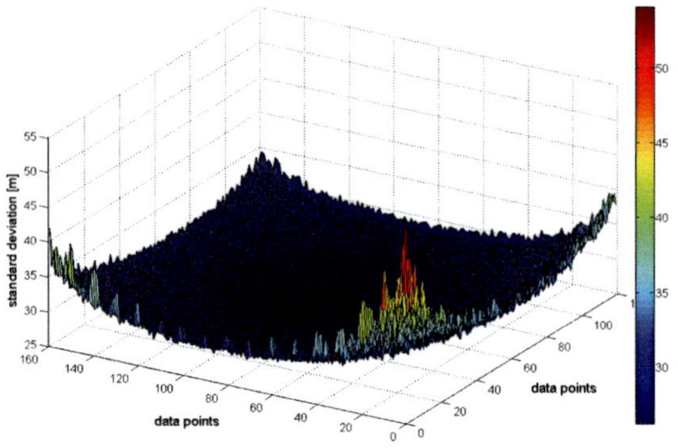

Figure 4.13: Depth data standard deviation of a depth image sequence that captured a homogeneously reflective and flat object for whole depth image data correction by using a point-illumination model of the TOF camera.

is used for correction which considers the TOF camera to be a point illumination source. This is valid because of the relatively small opening angle of 16° and a working distance greater than 2.0 m. The assumption is supported by figure 4.13 with its curved profile. It shows the standard deviation of a depth image sequence. The standard deviation which increases towards the image borders implies an increasing level of noise towards the image borders. Because a homogeneously reflective and flat object is considered, this characteristic implies that the distance to the object and, therefore, the illumination strength is the cause for this effect. The curved profile characteristic is approximately a sphere which supports the point illumination model of the TOF camera illumination for this purpose.

The proposed calibration technique was presented at the workshop *Time of Flight Camera based Computer Vision* which was held in conjunction with the *IEEE International Conference of Computer Vision and Pattern Recognition* and the VISAPP and published through [79] and [85], respectively.

Due the technical improvement of TOF cameras (e. g. the registered color channel and a increased resolution) another TOF camera was incorporated for the further development of the system. The described correction method represents important preliminary work for the data correction of the *3DVSystems ZCam*.

4.1.4.2 Incident Light Correction for the *ZCam*

Technical improvements of TOF cameras led to the decision to apply another TOF camera for the considered application . In spite of the technical improvements (e. g. the registered color channel and a increased resolution) systematic errors remained and depth data is not accurate enough to meet the requirements of the considered application of gait parameter determination. Therefore, depth errors must be calibrated out to meet the requirements. Because the *ZCam* is different to the *PMD [vision] 19k* with respect to its operating mode (see section 2.4.3), a proper correction has to be developed for the *ZCam* too.

As for the *PMD [vision] 19k* a data study proceeded the development of the depth data calibration for the *3DVSystems ZCam*. The data acquisition step was carried out in a similar way than for the *PMD [vision] 19k*. Therefore, it is not comprehensively described and just the differences are described.

Due to the smaller work space of the *3DVSystems ZCam*, a distance range between 2m and 3.5m with a variety of 14 targets with different reflectance property is considered for data evaluation. A subset of these 14 targets is shown in figure 4.14. The integration time is indirectly set for the *ZCam* by choosing a suited distance and width (see equation 2.7). Because the work space for the considered application of gait parameter determination ranges from 2m to 3.5m, the distance and width are set according to these prerequisites. Therefore, the integration time remains constant for this data acquisition.
The figure 4.15 displays the distance error for objects with different reflectivities against different nominal distances. It shows that different reflectivities affect the distance error. In general, it can be stated that the lower the reflectivities the bigger the distance error. When comparing the data for different nominal distances, a proportional dependence of

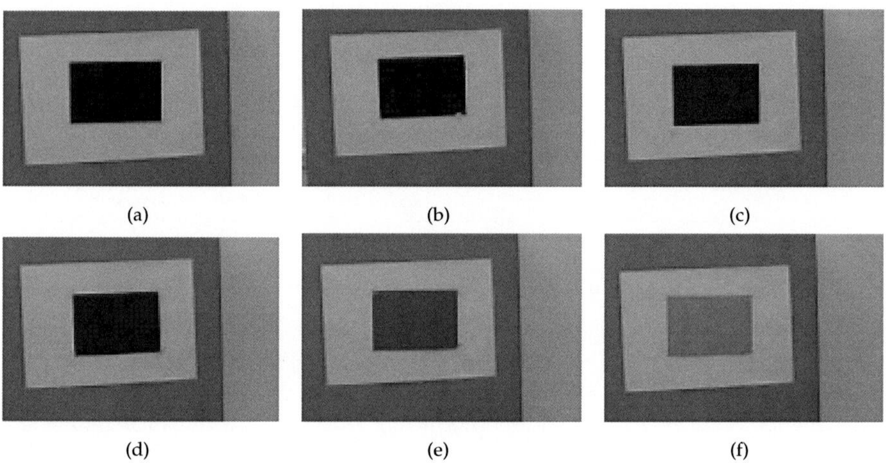

Figure 4.14: Subset of the 14 targets ($a - f$) used for investigations distinguished by their reflectance properties in the used IR-spectrum. The targets are ordered with respect to the distance offset they cause.

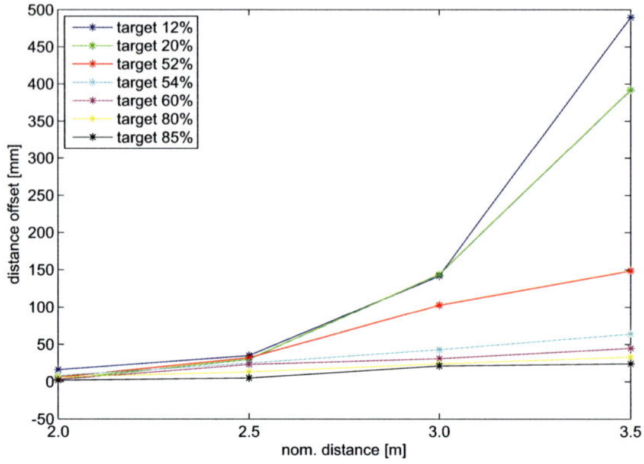

Figure 4.15: Distance error plotted against the nominal distance for targets with different reflectivities. It shows that the measured distances show an increasing drift for lower IR-reflectivities.

this offset $dist_{OS}$ in relation to the nominal distance $dist_n$ is noticed. Another specialty of the *ZCam* is the altered amount of noise that seems to be due to an interpolation of the low resoluted depth map to achieve higher resolutions, i. e., the *ZCam* captures the depth data at a lower resolution than the color image. These two images with different resolution are registered to each other through an interpolation of the depth data. The issue of noise reduction is faced in section 4.1.3. It is evident that the amount of noise, the reflectivities and the depth error are correlated in the way that a lower object's reflectivity results in altered noise which results in an increasing distance error towards erroneous bigger distance measurements. This knowledge is exploited for depth data correction.

Therefore, the main concept of the proposed method is the estimation of the reflectivity of the object and to use these estimations for depth correction. For this purpose first the noise from a single image is estimated. Thereby, the depth data correction incorporates an illumination modeling assuming a point illumination source to cope with illumination inhomogeneities for whole image data correction. To estimate the amount of noise from a single image one has to distinguish between noise and variations in the image yielded by the viewed scene. In this work a model is used which actually over-estimates the noise. The estimation is done by arithmetically subtracting an edge preserving bilateral filtered image with the original one. Since this model assumes additive noise and real camera (CCD) noise is not additive and strongly dependent on the intensities, there are regions in which the model does not hold. Nevertheless, this model yielded sufficient correct estimates for the considered application.

To reiterate, the data correction is achieved by incorporating a reflectivity estimate. The reflectivity is estimated on the base of a noise estimate and the intensity of the color image. This is achieved as follows.
The color image is illuminated through environmental lighting. Therefore, one has to assume diffuse light as mostly occurring indoors like in our application. Additionally, one has to keep in mind that the color image is captured on the base of the environmental light and, therefore, differs slightly in the bandwidth. Figure 4.14 demonstrates that these bandwidth differences are small since the objects are ordered according to their IR reflectivity and appear also ordered for visual-reflectivity.
To be able to distinguish between object's reflectivities and shades caused by the environmental light, the color intensity is considered together with the noise. To compensate for the illumination characteristic of the depth camera, the illumination characteristic is modeled by a point illumination source. For this purpose, a factor r and an additional scaling factor σ_2 are introduced. Here, r represents the Euclidean distance between the $\vec{x}$ and the optical center $\vec{x_{cp}} = (p_x, p_y)^T$ such that $r(x,y) = \sqrt{(x-p_x)^2 + (y-p_y)^2}$. The depth data correction is then achieved by the following equation:

$$\begin{aligned} D_c(x,y) &= D_m(x,y)|_{N(V_{NoiseEst})} + \\ &\quad \frac{V_{NoiseEst}}{V_{Refl}(x,y)+1} \cdot \sigma_1 + \\ &\quad r(x,y)^2 \cdot \sigma_2 \end{aligned}$$

This depth data correction consists of three parts.

The first part $D_m(x,y)|_{N(V_{NoiseEst})}$ is a smoothed value of local depth values in a neighborhood. The size of this neighborhood is computed by incorporating the reflectivity and the noise estimate. The computation pipeline of the neighborhood size is pseudo coded in algorithm 1. The computation of D_m, then, simple ends up in a local averaging to:

$$D_m(x,y) = \frac{1}{N} \sum^{N(V_{NoiseEst}, Region_{Refl})} D(x,y)$$

The second part of the equation is a reflectivity estimate. Here, higher values of the noise estimate indicate a lower reflectivity. Lower intensities of color also indicate lower reflectivities resulting in total in a reflectivity dependent factor which finally is scaled by σ_1.

Algorithm 1 The pseudo code below specify the neighborhood size N computation.

Init: $N_{max} \leftarrow 13$, $N_{min} \leftarrow 5$, $scale \leftarrow 0.4$
if $\|scale \cdot V_{NoiseEst}\| > N_{min})$ **then**
  $N \leftarrow \|scale \cdot V_{NoiseEst}\| \vee N_{max}$
  if $(!Nmod(2))$ **then**
    $N \leftarrow N + 1$
  end if
else
  $N \leftarrow N_{min}$
end if

The third part handles the lateral drift due to inhomogeneous illumination through the aforementioned distance from the optical center $r(x, y)$ which is scaled with σ_2 as a function of the squared depth. Here, the depth D_m is used for this purpose.

4.1.5 Flying Pixel Identification

The depth data represents the depth between an object and the TOF camera and can be seen as an objects' surface elevation profile. Because the currently common low resolutions of the TOF cameras, undersampling often occurs especially at discontinuities of the depth. Depth discontinuities refer to borders between objects that are at different distances to the camera. The effect of the undersampling is that at a depth discontinuity the distance measurement is based partly on the foreground object's distance and partly on the background object's distance. Therefore, the measured distance lies between the distances of both objects and represents neither of the distances correctly. Because the proportion between foreground and background distance is not known, these so-called *flying pixels* cannot be corrected without applying some model information and have to be identified and rejected. Figure 4.16 shows an example with the *flying pixels* between the two objects.

The identification of *flying pixel* is achieved through a variance filtering which is as a nonlinear edge detector. The analytical description of the filter at a position (x, y) in the depth image is given by the equation:

$$FPiD_{x,y} = \sigma_{x,y}^2 = \frac{1}{(2N+1)^2} \sum_{i=-N}^{+N} \sum_{j=-N}^{+N} (d_{x+i,y+j} - \bar{d}_{x,y})^2 \tag{4.13}$$

Here, $\bar{d}_{x,y}$ is the mean depth of the considered neighborhood N. The correction of the data is principally possible if information about the captured scene or additional data is

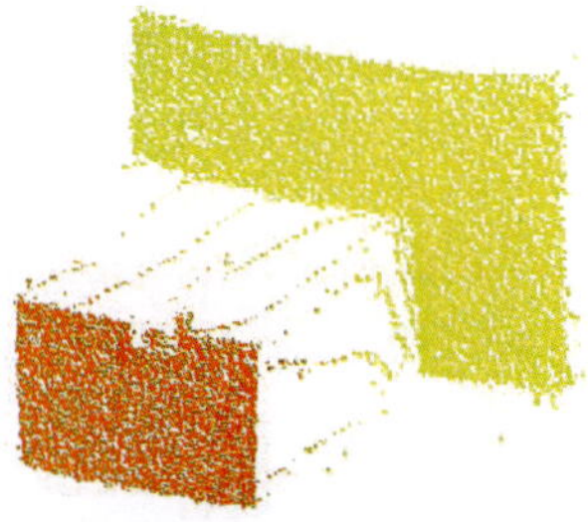

Figure 4.16: Occurrence of *flying pixels* at depth discontinuities. Due to lateral undersampling the *flying pixels* appear between the planar foreground object and the background. The foreground object is colored in orange whereas the background is yellow.

present. One example for a superresolution approach that also works with depth images captured with a TOF range imaging camera is [93]. The approach requires multiple depth images captured from slightly different views so that in this case additional data is present. This approach requires static sceneries without moving objects. Because we are capturing moving objects, such approaches are not appropriate. Additionally, because of the convex characteristics of the object, a correction of the data would be a demanding task and currently with the present noise not robust. Therefore, a correction of the *flying pixels* is not possible so that the *flying pixels* are discarded from 3D point cloud reconstruction.

4.2 Concept for Depth Data Based Gait Parameter Determination

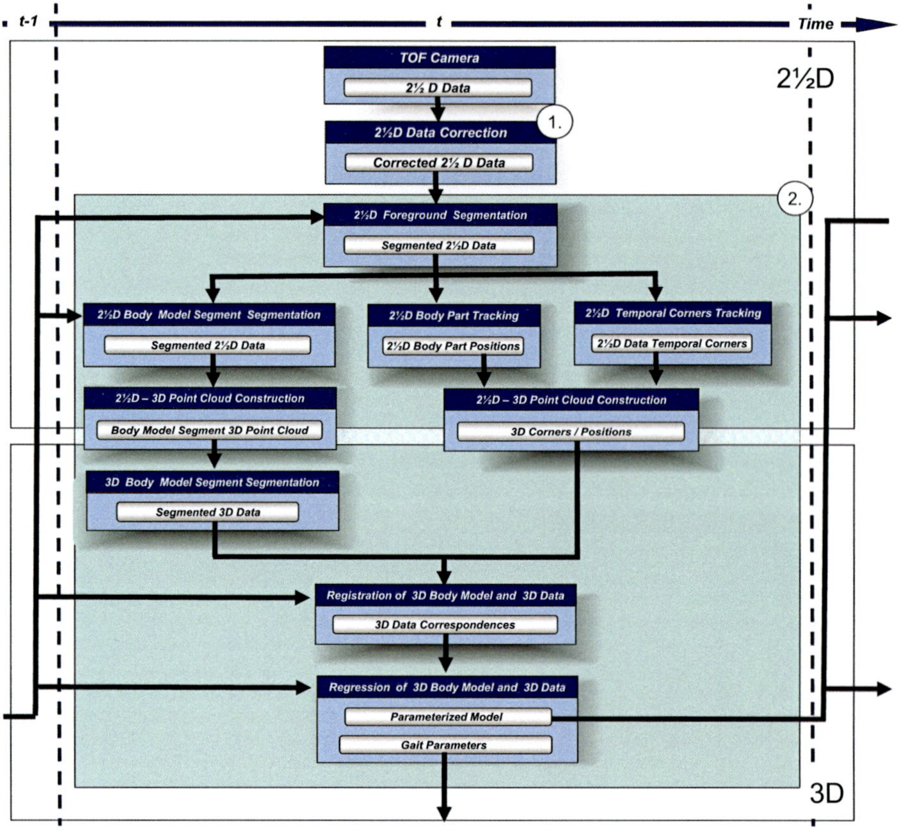

Figure 4.17: The processing pipeline from the TOF camera to the gait parameters of the realized system for subsequent frames with focus on gait parameter determination.

In this section the concept for the gait parameter determination is described. A flow chart of the processing pipeline for subsequent frames is given in figure 4.17. This flow chart is a more specified version of the overview flow chart from figure 4.1. The depth data correction marked with a ① is not specified because already covered by the previous section. The remaining processing stages in the flow chart compute the posture of the body model so that it corresponds to the posture of the captured human. They correspond to ② in the figure 4.1 and are described in the following.

The TOF camera provides the $2\frac{1}{2}$D data which at first is corrected as described in the previous section 4.1. The corrected $2\frac{1}{2}$D data are passed to the *foreground segmentation* processing stage in which the $2\frac{1}{2}$D data are segmented that represent the human body. The processing stage is carried out to coarsely reduce the amount of data for further processing (see section 4.2.5). Thereby, the parameterized model, which represents the determined posture of the human in the previous frame, is incorporated (see section 4.2.4). The foreground segmented data are handed to three further different processing stages; the *$2\frac{1}{2}$D body model segment segmentation*, the *$2\frac{1}{2}$D temporal corners tracking* and the *$2\frac{1}{2}$D body part tracking*:

1. Within the *$2\frac{1}{2}$D body model segment segmentation* processing stage the foreground segmented $2\frac{1}{2}$D data are further segmented with respect to the single body segments of the used 3D body model. For this purpose the parameterized model from the previous frame is incorporated in this processing stage also. The segmentation of the data with respect to the single body segments is important because it defines which data are used for which body segments in the final *regression* processing stage. The segmentation is performed in 2D image space on $2\frac{1}{2}$D data to be able to exploit local filters and to reduce the processing rate. The *$2\frac{1}{2}$D body model segment segmentation* processing stage is explained in section 4.2.6.
2. The *$2\frac{1}{2}$D body part tracking* processing stage counters sparse, unsecure 3D points within the *regression* processing stage. Such sparse data occurs at small body segments where the data are too sparse to be accurately corrected. The body part tracking is a non-parametric tracker adapted to the specifics of depth data. It is initialized through a skin-color segmentation for enhanced performance at the hands. It is explained in section 4.2.9
3. Within the *$2\frac{1}{2}$D temporal corners tracking* processing stage temporal corners are determined over several frames which enable the *regression* processing stage to cover rotations. This is not possible with standard regression approaches, but the measurement of rotation of the pelvis is a critical aspect of the development of a biomechanical analysis system. The description of the approach of temporal corners is described in section 4.2.8.

The resulting $2\frac{1}{2}$D data from these processing stages are projected into 3D for further processing (see section 4.1.1).
Because the segmentation in the *$2\frac{1}{2}$D body model segment segmentation* processing stage is performed in image space, occlusions can not be resolved. Therefore, these data points that were not segmented because they could not be assigned to a specific body segment are segmented in 3D within a postprocessing stage *3D body model segment segmentation*

(see section 4.2.6).
These data and the data from the $2\frac{1}{2}D$ *body part tracking* and the $2\frac{1}{2}D$ *temporal corners tracking* processing stage are handed over to the *registration* processing stage which is in the preparation of the 3D *regression* processing stage to determine the 3D model posture. The registration is performed through a closest point computation which is described in section 4.2.7.1. The 3D model based regression is described in section 4.2.7. Both processing stages together form the *iterative-closest-point* (ICP) and are carried out iteratively until convergence. Thereby, it should be noted that the segmentation processing stage is included in this iteration loop so that the segments newly determined for every iteration. This is not depicted for simplicity. The gait parameters are defined by the poses of the different body segments.
The work presented in this chapter were published by [81], [82], [83], [84].

4.2.1 Sensor View selection

When a single-view camera system is used, the question about the most appropriate view has to be answered. There are different views one can capture the human for the purpose of gait analysis. Two of them are interesting and will be discussed in the following. Both views have advantages and disadvantages.

Normally, only the movements along the sagittal plane are considered in gait analysis (see [75]). This suggests a capturing from the side when using a 2D camera. Another view becomes reasonable according to Hesse [41] (see section 2.2.2). The first and most important objective for gait rehabilitation is to regain gait symmetry, i. e., at first the sym-

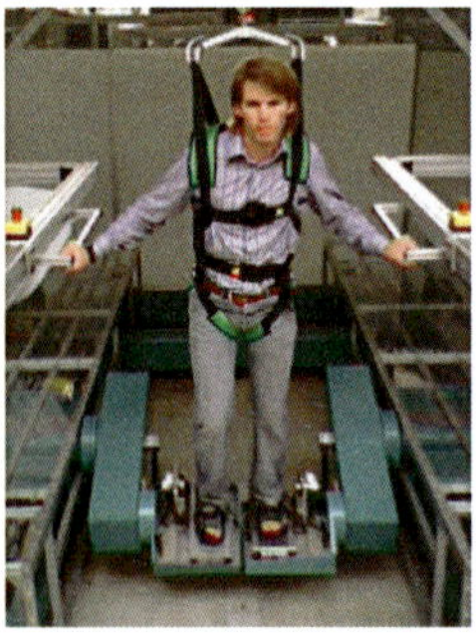

(a)

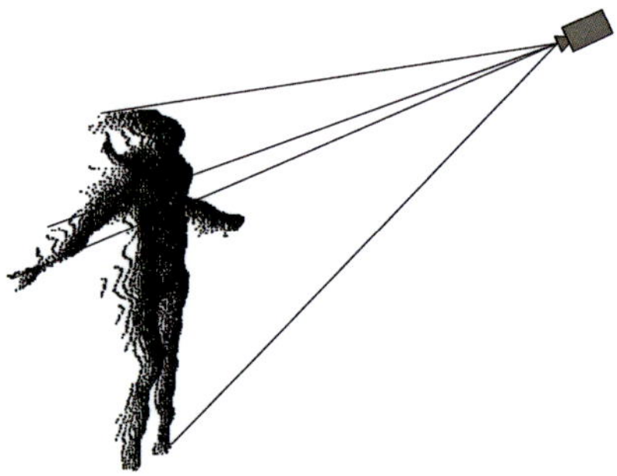

(b)

Figure 4.18: The image visualizes the chosen view of the TOF camera. (a) is a captured color image whereas (b) is the visualization of the 3D point cloud reconstructed from the corrected depth data, the TOF camera and a few exemplary lines of sights.

metric weight takeover because this is a fundamental base for further progresses. This gait feature is best captured from the front or back, respectively. The sagittal movements are represented by the depth data and therefore are also captured from this view.

In this thesis the frontal view is selected for capturing. This has two main reasons: The first reason is the importance of the gait symmetry which is best captured from the front. The second reason is of a technical perspective. The frontal aspect of the human shows less occlusions, especially at the legs. This has the simple background that occlusions represent a loss of data which needs to be compensated for the determination of the body model posture somehow. Therefore, the frontal view provides a more stable base for a accurate gait parameter determination.
The TOF camera is hinged at a height of 2.2 meters to not obstruct the area in front of the gait rehabilitation robot *HapticWalker*. The figure 4.18 (a) shows an example image of the chosen view whereas figure 4.18 (b) is the visualization of the 3D point cloud constructed from the captured depth data, the TOF camera and some exemplary lines of sight.

4.2.2 Concept for Comparison of 3D Human Body and $2\frac{1}{2}$D Data

Because the human body is three dimensional and TOF cameras just provide a $2\frac{1}{2}$D projection of the scene, the question needs to be answered:

- How to compare the $2\frac{1}{2}$D data and 3D features of the human body?

There are two concepts for a comparison:

1. One is to project the 3D features of the human body into $2\frac{1}{2}$D data space and to perform the comparison in $2\frac{1}{2}$D then.
2. The other concept is to reproject the $2\frac{1}{2}$D data from the TOF camera to 3D space and compare it in 3D space with the 3D features of the human body.

In the first concept the projection of the 3D human body features into $2\frac{1}{2}$D implies a scaling which leads to non-linear equations. This is due to the perspective projection of the TOF camera. Therefore the distance metric for the comparison of the 3D features and the $2\frac{1}{2}$D data varies with the distance of the 3D object to the camera.
In the second concept 3D data is projectively reconstructed of the $2\frac{1}{2}$D so that these problems do not occur. But this concept suffers from non uniform distance measures in 3D and $2\frac{1}{2}$D space. This means that the relation of the distances between two reconstructed 3D points and the distances between the corresponding pixels in the projective $2\frac{1}{2}$D range image varies according to the distance to the camera projection center.

In this work the second concept is followed. The reason for choosing this concept is that the gait parameters are three dimensional and for an iterative determination of the gait parameters the $2\frac{1}{2}$D data just need to be transformed to 3D once for each frame and can directly be compared to the 3D features of the body. With the first concept the 3D gait parameters need to be transformed to $2\frac{1}{2}$D for each iteration. Therefore, the first concept is less computational expensive which is more favorable for reaching real-time performance.

4.2.3 Concept for Depth Data Representation

Sensor and sensor view were selected to provide a proper sensory base for the considered application. The next step is to evaluate and select a representation of the data so that the data processing can be carried out in an efficient and effective way. There are two representations of depth data that are interesting for this work. These are:

- $2\frac{1}{2}$D Panoramic Image (Depth-color panorama)
  A $2\frac{1}{2}$*D panoramic image* which is also called depth map encodes depth in a 2D representation. This can be done, e. g., in planar, cylindrical or spherical coordinates. A more general representation of this is the $2\frac{1}{2}$*D layered depth image* such that it wraps multiple registered depth images in one representation. This means that for every pixel multiple measurements are stored. This enables the layered depth image to represent dynamics and occlusions separately.
- Unstructured 3D Point Clouds
  The *unstructured 3D point cloud* can be generated from depth data by applying equation 4.4 together with the equations 2.3 for the *PMD [vision] 19k* or the equation 2.7 for the *ZCam*, respectively. The 3D point cloud representation is not dependent on the distance from the camera because it is not based on a central perspective. On the other hand this representation does not provide any neighboring relations. Therefore, the realization of local filters in 3D is a demanding task.

Both representations have specific advantages and disadvantages in different situations. Therefore, both representations shall be used such that dependent on the situation the most appropriate one is taken.
The major advantage of the $2\frac{1}{2}$*D panoramic image* representation is the ability to represent neighboring relations. This is important if, e. g., local filters need to be applied. This is the case for noise reduction or non trivial foreground segmentation. Additionally, most existing image processing routines can easily be adapted for depth data processing or directly applied.

The *unstructured 3D point cloud* representation is chosen also because it directly represents the 3D space and not just a projection of it, like the $2\frac{1}{2}D$ *panoramic image* representation does due to the camera inherent central perspective. Therefore, the model needs not to be rescaled dependent on the distance from the TOF camera. See section 4.2.2 for the related discussion.

4.2.4 3D Human Body Model

The motivation for the use of body models is to use knowledge about the human body for the tracking and, hence, to reduce the degrees of freedom (DOF) for the posture determination process.
As mentioned in section 4.2.2 the 3D human model is parameterized by a comparison of the 3D point cloud and the 3D body model. Because this procedure comprises first a synthesis of the posture of the model and then an analysis of that posture, it is referred to as an analysis-by-synthesis approach. In this context the 3D model practically presents an articulated reference for the comparison of the reconstructed 3D point cloud and the 3D model. Crucial for the design of the model is that the degrees of freedom of the model should be adjusted according to application's needs. A reduction of the degrees of freedom narrows the flexibility but also reduces the computational load. Thus, the number of degrees of freedom varies a lot in existing works. For example up to 50 degrees of freedom are considered in [1].

Models used for human motion capturing represent the kinematic structure of the human as well as its dimensions. The kinematic structure is described as a kinematic tree or skeleton, respectively, whose parts are connected by joints. These joints should be adapted to the physiology of the human. This is achieved by limiting, e. g., the joint angles, the joint velocities or the joint accelerations [102], [106] as well as the space the body parts can occupy. In this thesis just the joint angles are limited because this already provides reasonable results as shall be seen in the results section. This is due to the small movements performed by the humans. There are different concepts for joint modeling, such as [19], [26], [49], [69], whereat [49] is adapted within this work.
The kinematic tree often refers to a rigid-body-model. That means that the body segments are represented by rigid elements. In this context one has to keep in mind that at a certain acceleration the rigid body assumption is not valid any more. This is due to the inhomogeneous consistency of the human body with its soft tissues, muscles and bones which move increasingly independent with increasing acceleration [40], [56]. Since in this thesis gait movements with minor velocity and acceleration are considered, this artifact

is neglected, especially when considering gait in rehabilitation scenario with impaired patients.

Human body models exist in 2D and 3D. The 3D models are defined either by volume or surface representation describing a volume. A classic variant is the *Constructive Solid Geometry* (CSG)-model which consists of single body segments representing volume entities. This is actually a further development of the 2D *Cardboard*-models ([7],[45]) to 3D. In this context two questions appear:

- How to partition the body into single segments according to the requirements of the considered application?
- How to properly describe the body segments, i. e., the volume or the surfaces, respectively?

The first question about the partitioning can be reformulated as the determination of the relevant joints between the body segments. For this reason the normal gait and the abnormal gait of patients after stroke with their specific pathologic patterns was examined in order to determine the relevant joints and their degree of freedom. An essay on human gait in general and of patients after stroke is given in section 2.2.
The body model resulting from this examination consists of 11 body parts which are arranged in a hierarchical way. The partitioning and its hierarchy are displayed in figure 4.19(a). In this figure the hierarchy is illustrated trough different intensities of the background of the related segment. The higher the intensity the higher the hierarchy level. Within this hierarchy the torso presents the root. The origin of the body model

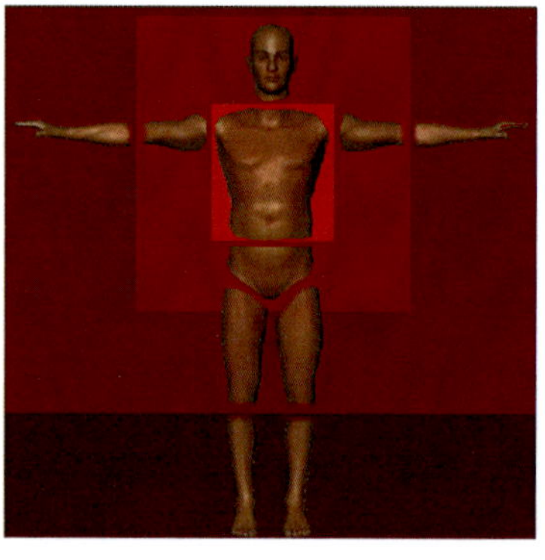

(a)

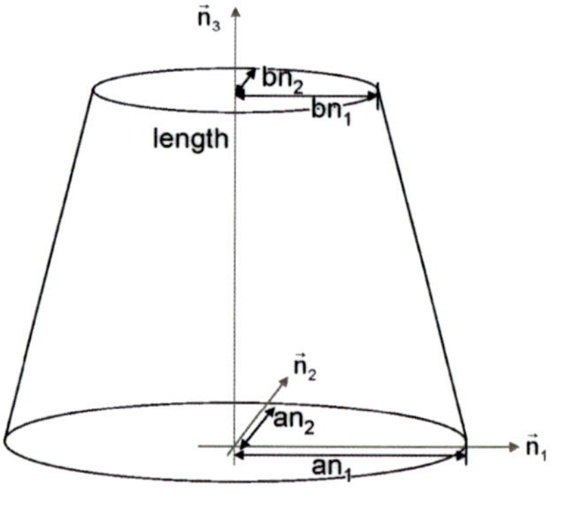

(b)

Figure 4.19: (a) shows the partitioning of the model used for this thesis. The different color intensities represent the hierarchy of the model segments. (b) shows a generalized truncated cone to represent the body segments.

coordinate system is located at the lower torso to the pelvis for whole body translation and rotation. From the torso the other body parts branch out in a sequential way, i. e. the 'upper arms', the 'thighs' and the 'head' belong to the second level of hierarchy. The remaining body parts belong to the third level. 19 joints connect the body segments across the hierarchy levels and, thereby, configure the underlying sequential kinematic structure of the body model. The joint between torso and pelvis, the neck, the shoulders and the hip joints are parameterized by three DOF. Elbow and knee are modeled as hinged joints with one DOF.

The second question concerns the volume representation which is closely related to the used regression method which in our case is based on the Euclidean distances between model and 3D point (see section 4.2.7). Many model volume descriptions exist, such as the advanced triangulated mesh model with 46 DOF or the less complex model descriptions with e. g. cylindrical models [2]. In [4] the triangulated mesh model and the cylindrical model are compared for evaluation. Thereby, it has emerged that the less complex cylindrical model performed better in terms of precision (i. e., estimated model silhouette overlap of foreground) with 91.07 % but slightly fails in recall (i. e., explain the foreground by the model) with 75.12 %. Thereby, it should be noted that the model is learned from a volume scan of the person for which reason it seems much more adequate to use a model representation which is not based on a previous volumetric body scan. Because of this and the only slight inferiority of the cylindrical model in comparison with the sophisticated triangulated mesh model, in this work the body segment surface is modeled by a generalized truncated cone (see figure 4.19(b)) which is similar to the cylindrical model. It can be described by a simple mathematical function. As in [49] the segments are parameterized by the four radii for the both base ellipsis an_1, an_2 and bn_1, bn_2 and the length (see figure 4.19(b)).

4.2.5 Foreground Segmentation

The foreground segmentation is the first processing stage after depth data correcion. See figure 4.17 for overview over the processing stages and their interaction.

Image segmentation generally plays a crucial role in many image processing applications. It deals with the partitioning of an image into several regions or segments. Therefore, it is an important preprocessing stage to facilitate subsequent processing steps or to increase the overall performance of the application. In the ideal case, the subsequent processing steps simplify to such an extent that they become trivial or completely vanish.
In this work, the segmentation aims at segmenting the human body as foreground so that further processing only is performed on the segmented data. This avoids the com-

putational expensive regression with 3D data points that do not belong to the captured human.

Generally, for any segmentation it is problematic when the image features, such as the gray value of the pixels, have a low discriminatory power level. For example, if several objects have similar colors, segmentation becomes more difficult as if the discriminatory power levels were high. This normally leads to a lower quality of the segmentation results. This is the case for e. g. the legs because the color of the trouser legs is usually equal or very similar for both legs. Moreover, it is possible that the color of the clothes corresponds to the background. An example of such a scenario is shown in figure 4.20(a). Segmentation only on the base of color might lead to an erroneous segmentation as displayed in figure 4.20(b). Here, parts of the foreground (the lower legs) and the background (the floor) are segmented as if they were one segment. A characteristic of physical objects is that they are contiguous in depth. Depth data provides this information so that it is exploited for segmentation.

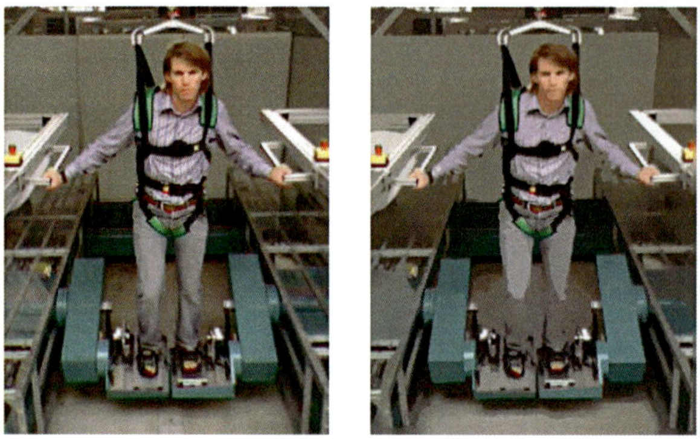

(a) (b)

Figure 4.20: (a) shows an example of a to be segmented image and (b) shows the possible result of a color segmentation where the lower parts of the trousers are erroneously assigned to the same segment as the floor.

The *floodfill*-method is ideally suited for this because it just considers only a part of the data and is capable for combining different data [38]. *Floodfill* is a function which is often used to isolate parts of an image according to the similarity of neighboring pixels emerging from *seed points*. These seed points have to be selected in advance. The processing pipeline for the foreground segmentation results into a four stage process:

1. determine *seed points*.
2. compensate view inclination angle.

3. apply *floodfill* method on corrected depth.
4. post process, i. e., fill holes, discard small blobs.

Important parameters of the *floodfill* are the measure of *similarity* S within the neighborhood as well as the *termination criterion* and the already described determination of the *seed points*. These parameters and the seed point determination are explained in the following.

First, the *seed points* are determined. Due to the inclined camera the closest points refer to the head and torso (see figure 4.21(a)). These closest points are taken as *seed points*. The closest points are determined by taking the pixels of 1-percentile minimum distance.

Second, to be able to set the *termination criterion* of the *floodfill* as tight as possible the inclination angle of the TOF camera is compensated for foreground segmentation (see figure 4.21 for visualization). Actually, this perspective transformation needs to be carried out in 3D, but since in 3D the neighboring relations are lost, a 2D approximation of the perspective is used. A perspective transform in 3D and a subsequent projection would result in a depth image with regions without depth data or with ambiguous depths. Therefore, the 2D approximation is chosen. The perspective deformations of the 2D approximation are insignificant because the approximation is just used for foreground object mask determination.

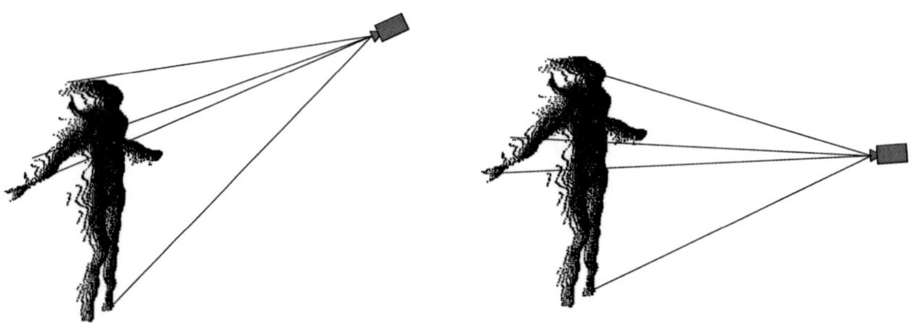

(a) (b)

Figure 4.21: (a) visualizes the chosen view of the TOF range imaging camera (see section 4.2.1). From this perspective of the camera the foreground object covers a bigger depth range as if the camera would be placed in front of the human without any inclination. For foreground segmentation it is desirable reduce the depth range that is covered by the body and, therefore, to compensate for this perspective deformation such as visualized in (b).

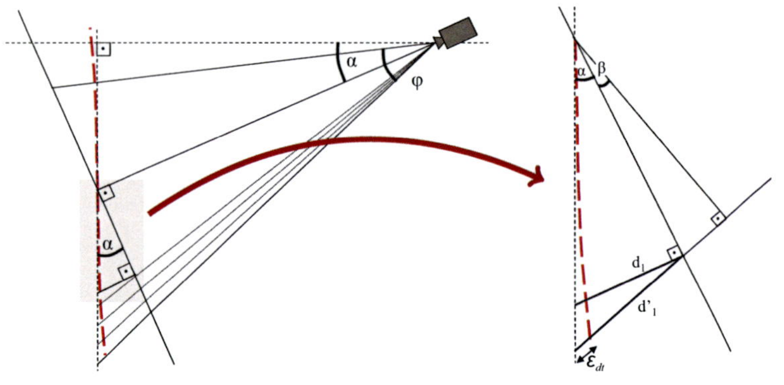

(a) (b)

Figure 4.22: (a) 2D perspective transformation approximation to compensate for the camera inclination. The depth data is transformed according to its position in the depth image. Here, φ is the opening angle and α is the inclination angle of the camera. The red line illustrates the absolute error $\epsilon_{d_t}(\alpha, \beta)$. The drawing (b) zooms into the gray region of (a) in which the real (d_1') and the approximated (d_1) depths are marked.

With α being the inclination angle of the TOF-camera, the depth data d is transformed to $d_t = d + y \cdot tan(\alpha) - offset$. Here, a constant offset of 50 yields reasonable results. This transformation includes a depth error ϵ_{d_t} which is less than 8% and assumes a vertical object. With this the depth error can be estimated with $\beta_{max} = \frac{\varphi}{2}$:

$$\epsilon_{d_t}(\alpha, \beta) < \epsilon_{d_t max}(\alpha, \frac{\varphi}{2}) \lesssim \frac{cos\frac{\varphi}{2} \cdot cos(\alpha + \frac{\varphi}{2}) - sin\frac{\varphi}{2}}{cos\alpha} \quad (4.14)$$

This error is not critical since the compensation of the depth data is only used to determine the foreground and no further processing is carried out with the transformed depth data. The 2D perspective transform approximation is visualized in figure 4.22. Here, the transformed depth d_t including the error $\epsilon_{d_t}(\alpha, \beta)$ is drawn as a red colored dashed line.

Third, the *floodfill* is performed. This requires the definition of a similarity measure and a termination criterium.

The measure of similarity S between a cluster pixel a with value v_a and a neighboring candidate pixel b with value v_b is defined as:

$$S(a, b) = \|\mu_a - d_b\| \quad (4.15)$$

μ_a represents the median value of the clustered 8 neighborhood of pixel a. As termination criterion a lower lo and an upper hi bound of this similarity measure is set to $lo = 35$ and $hi = 25$, respectively, so that a candidate pixel b is marked as foreground FG according

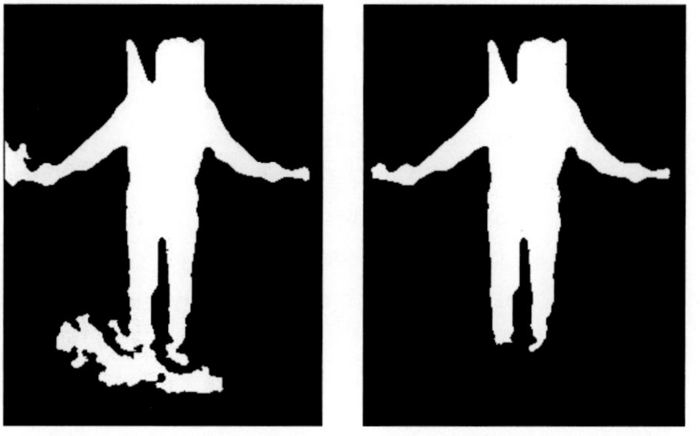

(a) (b)

Figure 4.23: (a) illustrates the problem of an erroneous segmentation which is based on depth data only if the foreground object is in contact with other objects. This is due to the sole exploitation of the spatial connectivity of an object. (b) foreground segmentation result of the same frame, when depth and color data is incorporated.

to:

$$\{a \in FG, S(a,b) \leq lo|_{\mu_a \geq v_b}, S(a,b) \leq hi|_{v_b \geq \mu_a}\} \rightarrow \{b \in FG\} \tag{4.16}$$

If just the depth data is considered for segmentation, the segmented foreground object might include parts of objects that are in contact with the actual foreground object. This is the case for the feet and the hands so that parts of the gait rehabilitation robot *HapticWalker* are segmented as foreground object. An example of this case is shown in figure 4.23(a). Therefore, both the color and the depth data are considered for segmentation.

The selection of the appropriate color space for this concern is mainly driven by the requirement that the color space should be uniform. *CIE L*a*b** is such a uniform color space which provides Euclidean distance between colors by nonlinear transformation [66]. The popular HSI color space is less suited for our purpose since being unstable at low saturations. The color and the depth data are combined by different scaling. Thereby, the depth data is adjusted to the color data with respect to its noise level which is estimated by a high pass-filter, analogous to the depth data enhancement (see page 61).

The incorporation of color and depth at the same time yielded improved foreground segmentation. The intermediate foreground segmentation result is shown in figure 4.23(b) which is post processed afterwards, i. e., some morphological functions are applied, e. g., to close holes or suppress the *flying pixels* (see section 4.1.5).

4.2.6 Body Model Segmentation of the Depth Data

The 3D body model consists of several body segments. To perform the regression of these body model segments only with the points that really represent this body model segment in the depth data frame, the points need to be segmented with respect to the corresponding body model segment. The process for this is described within this section. The assignment of the $2\frac{1}{2}$D data points to a specific body model segment can be done either in 3D or in 2D-image space.

- In 3D space the three dimensional distances between the body segments and the 3D points can be used as a measure for segmentation. This means that a 3D point is assigned to the body segment which is closest in three dimensional space.
- In 2D-image space the 3D model is projected into the depth data image and the lateral 2D distances in image space are used.

The difference between both strategies is that in the former strategy the $2\frac{1}{2}$D data must be transformed from 2D-image space to 3D point clouds, whereas in the latter strategy the model is transformed from 3D to 2D-image space. Both of these strategies have their specific advantages and disadvantages.

- The 3D approach allows for a coherent assignment when body segments are partially overlapping, but it is computational very expensive. This is because the 3D distances between each 3D point and all body segments have to be computed which results in the high computational load. The use of less computational expensive bounding boxes for the assignment suffers from intersecting bounding boxes of close body segments. An example for this is formed by the legs whose proximity results in an unstable ambiguous segmentation.
- The 2D approach, in contrast, performs the assignment in a more efficient way. Here, the depth data is assigned to the body segments according to their closest distance in 2D image space. This is computational less expensive because the computation is performed in 2D than in 3D with its additional dimension. However, it suffers when segments are overlapping. This is always the case at the contact regions of physiologically connected body segments.

Because both approaches are not able to cover all occurring cases, a combined strategy is followed. First the 2D approach is followed which covers more than 90% of the data. For the remaining points the 3D approach is applied. This guarantees an efficient assignment of the data while coping with the deficits of the 2D approach.

The segmentation with the 2D strategy works as follows. It is to be distinguished between three cases that are defined by the projection of the 3D body model into the depth data as shown in figure 4.24(a). The figures 4.24 (b)-(d) correspond to the different cases which are:

1. no body segment data (figure 4.24(b))
2. single body segment data (figure 4.24(c))
3. multiple body segment data (figure 4.24(d))

In the following the different cases are explained and with which strategy they will be approached.

CASE 1 (NO BODY SEGMENT DATA)

The case is defined by the fact that the projected model is not covering any depth data (see figure 4.24(b)). This case is addressed with the second 2D strategy because for this case it is important to assign the depth data to the body model segment which is closest. This can be done much more efficient in 2D than in 3D as already mentioned. For this purpose, a distance transform is applied which determines the lateral 2D distances emerging from the single projected body limbs [10]. Here, as distance metrics the *L2*-norm with $\rho(r) = r^2/2$ (r is the Euclidean distance) is used. The distance transformation and the final assignment for this case are shown in figure 4.25. Assigning the data to the single limbs of the body is difficult, i. e., unstable where segments join, especially, when the body shape appears concave, e. g., at the axles and the crotch. Therefore, in this sub

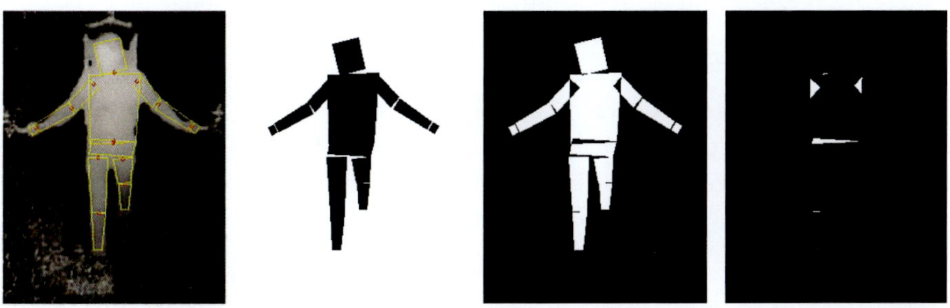

(a) (b) (c) (d)

Figure 4.24: Examples for all three cases of the body model segmentation. (a) is the depth data with the projected model. In (b) the region are marked white in which the line of sight of the corresponding depth data pixel does not pass any limb segment of the reprojected model whereas in (c) only those regions are white in which only one limb segment is passed. (d) displays the third case in which the line of sight passes through more than one limb.

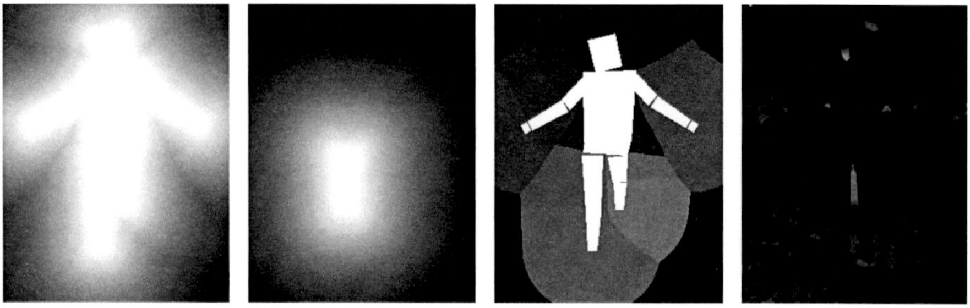

(a) (b) (c) (d)

Figure 4.25: These images display the different intermediate results of CASE 1. (a) shows the distance transform of the whole projected body model. This distance transform is compared with the distance transform for every single body model segment. (b) displays an example distance transform for the left thigh. Figure (c) shows the results of the assignment. The different shades of gray represent the regions assigned to the closest body segment. (d) is an intermediate result to mark out regions which are unstable and ambiguous in terms of the assignment.

case the depth data is not assigned. These concave body regions are detected with a 7×7 *blackhat* filter applied on the depth data (see figure 4.25(d)).

CASE 2 (SINGLE BODY SEGMENT DATA)

This case is defined by depth data that is covered by only one projected body segment (see figure 4.24(c)). The depth data is directly assigned to the according body limb. Because the movements of the subject take place mainly in the sagittal plane and are small in the frontal plane for each frame, the lateral movements are intrinsically compensated by the subsequent registration procedure. This is also valid for CASE 1 and could have been achieved by a motion detection method, such as the one published by us in [80], though simple frame difference image analysis would also work.

CASE 3 (MULTIPLE BODY SEGMENT DATA)

This case is defined by depth data which is covered by more than one body segment (see figure 4.24(d)). It is addressed by a 3D strategy that uses bounding boxes in 3D. As can be seen in figure 4.24(d) only a few points mostly belong to this category.

4.2.7 Registration and Regression of 3D Model and 3D Data

The registration process aligns the 3D model and the 3D point cloud and, therefore, represents a central part of the determination of the gait parameters. In the considered case of gait rehabilitation after stroke just little movements take place. Under the additional assumption that an initial pose is present, the registration can be carried out through a fine registration method. There are several fine registration methods, such as the *Iterative Closest Point* (ICP) [6] *genetic algorithms* or *Chen's method* [18] among others. A comprehensive survey of existing registration methods is given in [91]. These methods generally perform a minimization of a distance function.

From the mass of the registration methods the ICP method was selected. This has two main reasons. First, it was shown that the ICP method yields robust results, even for articulated objects [19], [26], [27], [49], [69], [70]. Second, according to [91], it is suited for real-time registration. In this thesis the approach of [49] is applied.

The ICP method was introduced by Besl and McKay [6]. It is still under research which yields many recent variations of it. The main idea is to minimize the distance between two point clouds on the base of point correspondences between these two point clouds. For this purpose, first the point clouds are transformed into a common reference system. The ICP computes the translation $\vec{t}$ and the rotation $\mathbf{R}$ to match the two point clouds $\mathcal{M} = \{\vec{m}_N, ..., \vec{m}_i, ..., \vec{m}_2, \vec{m}_1\}$ and $\mathcal{P} = \{\vec{p}_N, ..., \vec{p}_i, ..., \vec{p}_2, \vec{p}_1\}$ in 3D. Both point clouds have the same number N of elements. Here, P is the 3D point cloud reconstructed of the $2\frac{1}{2}$D data. The other 3D point cloud $\mathcal{M}$ is synthesized from the 3D model surface (see section 4.2.7.1). $\vec{m}_i$ and $\vec{p}_i$ refer to the i-th closest point pairs $\mathcal{CP}_i = \{\vec{p}_i, \vec{m}_i\}$.
The ICP steps are:

1. Determine corresponding closest points $\mathcal{CP}_i$ by the nearest neighbor criterion.
2. Estimate transformation (translation $\vec{t}$ and rotation $\mathbf{R}$) by minimizing a mean squared error cost function.
3. Transform the model according to the estimated transformation.
4. Iterate steps $1-3$ until a termination criterion (convergence or maximum number of iterations) is fulfilled.
5. iterate steps $1-4$ for all model segments according to model segment hierarchy.

The critical part of the registration process in terms of computational load is the determination of the point correspondences $\mathcal{CP}_i$ and the synthesis of the point cloud $\mathcal{M}$. The ICP method takes the closest Euclidean distance as measure to solve this correspondence problem as might be guessed from the method's name. The mean squared distances between the corresponding closest points are minimized (see eq. 4.17). This is performed iteratively until convergence. The computation process for synthesizing the point cloud $\mathcal{M}$ and determining the point correspondences $\mathcal{CP}_i$ is explained in section 4.2.7.1. There are different approaches to carry out the minimization based on, e. g., *singular value decompo-*

sition (SVD) or quaternion representation of the rotation. Both approaches are comparable in the complexity of the computation [47]. Here, the quaternion approach is taken.

$$f(\mathbf{R},\vec{t}) = \frac{1}{N}\sum_{i=1}^{N} \left\| m_i - \mathbf{R}(\vec{q_R})p_i - \vec{t} \right\|^2 \tag{4.17}$$

Here, $\vec{q_R} = [q_0, q_1, q_2, q_3]^T$ expressed in quaternions is the unit eigenvector which corresponds to the maximum eigenvalue of the symmetric matrix $\mathbf{Q}$ which is defined to minimize equation 4.17 [6].

$$\mathbf{Q}(\mathbf{\Sigma_{p,m}}) = \begin{bmatrix} trace(\mathbf{\Sigma_{p,m}}) & \Delta^T \\ \Delta^T & \mathbf{\Sigma_{p,m}} + \mathbf{\Sigma_{p,m}}^T - trace(\mathbf{\Sigma_{p,m}})I_3 \end{bmatrix} \tag{4.18}$$

Here, $\mathbf{\Sigma_{p,m}}$ is the cross-covariance matrix of $\mathcal{P}$ and $\mathcal{M}$, $\Delta = [A_{23}A_{31}A_{12}]$ is computed from a anti-symmetric matrix $A_{uv} = (\mathbf{\Sigma_{p,m}} - \mathbf{\Sigma_{p,m}}^T)_{uv}$. $\mathbf{\Sigma_{p,m}}$ is given by:

$$\mathbf{\Sigma_{p,m}} = \frac{1}{N}\sum_{i=1}^{N} [\vec{p_i}\vec{m_i}^T] - \vec{\mu_p}\vec{\mu_m}^T \tag{4.19}$$

On the base of $\vec{q_R}$ first the rotation $\mathbf{R}$ (eq. 4.20) and then the translation $\vec{t}$ (eq. 4.21) are computed by:

$$\mathbf{R} = \begin{bmatrix} q_0^2 + q_1^2 - q_2^2 - q_3^2 & 2(q_1q_2 - q_0q_3) & 2(q_1q_3 + q_0q_2) \\ 2(q_1q_2 - q_0q_3) & q_0^2 - q_1^2 + q_2^2 - q_3^2) & 2(q_2q_3 - q_1q_0) \\ 2(q_1q_3 + q_0q_2) & 2(q_2q_3 - q_1q_0) & q_0^2 - q_1^2 - q_2^2 + q_3^2 \end{bmatrix} \tag{4.20}$$

$$\vec{t} = \vec{\mu_m} - \mathbf{R}\vec{\mu_p} \tag{4.21}$$

4.2.7.1 Registration of 3D Model and 3D Data through Closest Point Computation

The computation of the closest point $\mathcal{CP}_i$ is illustrated in figure 4.26. Since the computation of the closest point $\vec{m_i}$ on the model of the 3D point $\vec{p_i}$ is one of the most computational intensive parts of the program, it is performed on the base of a perpendicular projection of the 3D point $\vec{p_i}$ with reference to the longitudinal orientation of the model segment similar to [49]. This guarantees a faster distance computation. The projection of $\vec{p_i}$ onto the model segment is described by the following equations. First the radii r_{cp1} and r_{cp2} are interpolated from the base ellipse parameters an_1, an_2, bn_1, bn_2, the truncated cone length *length* and $\vec{p_i}$'s local unit coordinates $[p_{il1}, p_{il2}, p_{il3}]^T$ with $\|\vec{p_{il}}\| = 1$ by:

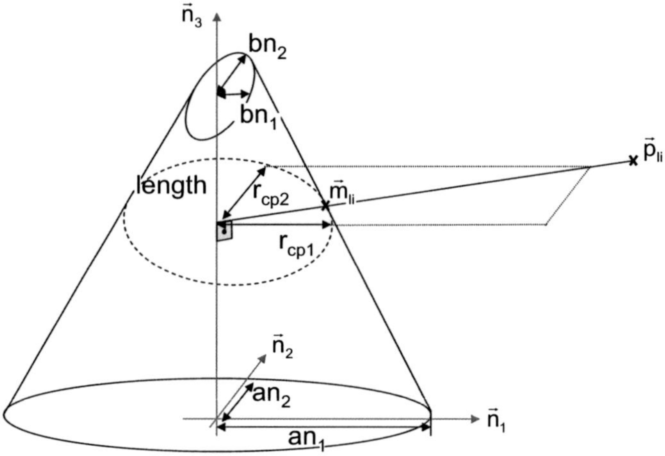

Figure 4.26: Closest point computation between the generalized truncated cone and 3D point $\vec{p_{il}}$.

$$r_{cp1} = \frac{bn_1 - an_1}{length} \cdot p_{il3} + an_1 \quad (4.22)$$
$$r_{cp2} = \frac{bn_2 - an_2}{length} \cdot p_{il3} + an_2$$

The corresponding point m_i of p_i is computed in body segment's local coordinates by the following equation. The algebraic sign is determined according to the related quadrant.

$$\vec{m}_i = \begin{bmatrix} m_{il1} \\ m_{il2} \\ m_{il3} \end{bmatrix} = \begin{bmatrix} \sqrt{\frac{r_{cp1}^2 \cdot r_{cp2}^2}{r_{cp2}^2 + (p_{il2}/p_{il1})^2 \cdot r_{cp1}^2}} \\ \frac{p_{il2}}{p_{il1}} \cdot m_{il1} \\ p_{il3} \end{bmatrix} \quad (4.23)$$

It happens that 3D points are inside or behind of the generalized truncated cone. This is due to movements away from the camera. The figure 4.27 shows this situation where the camera is depicted on the left side. The model whose pose was determined in the previous frame (t-1) is visualized as a red circle. The $2\frac{1}{2}$D data profile of the current frame (t) is represented by the black solid line on the right. The vertical parts of that line correspond to a flat background (e. g. a wall) whilst the part towards the camera is the curved object. In this situation the closest point is not the actual corresponding point of the 3D point on the model surface. This normally results in an increased number of ICP iterations, at first the wrong corresponding point is taken.

When the object moves away from the camera, the 3D point is behind the model from the

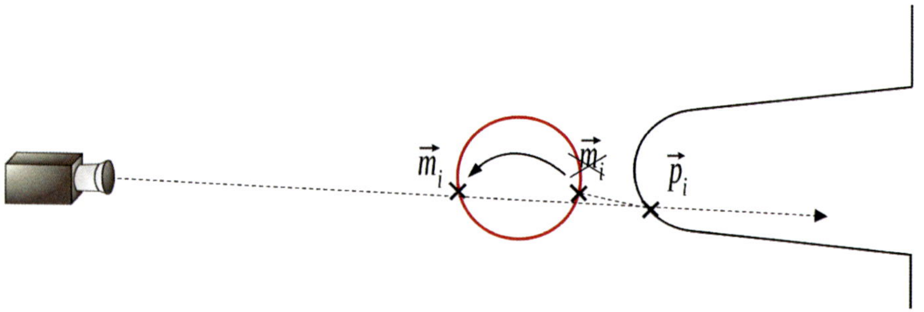

Figure 4.27: Correction of the closest point for the first iterations to reduce the number of ICP-iterations. It happens that at the first iterations the closest point is not the correct corresponding point. Therefore, the corresponding point $\vec{m}_i$ of a point $\vec{p}_i$, that lies behind or within the model (from camera's view), is determined by projecting it to the front side of the model.

camera's view. When the corresponding point on the model $\vec{m}_i$ is determined by means of the closest distance between point $\vec{p}_i$ and the model, the corresponding point $\vec{m}_i$ on the model lies on the back of the model (from the camera's view).
Because $2\frac{1}{2}$D data represents the front surface of the captured object, the corresponding point pair that are determined by means of the closest distance are far from the correct corresponding points. To compensate for this effect, an additional stage for corresponding point correction is introduced. Within this stage, the points that are behind or in the back part of the model are projected to the front surface of the model (from camera's view point). This effectuates that the number of ICP-iterations is reduced, when the object moves away from the camera. At the end of the ICP iteration when the ICP converges, the model and the depth data profile are already close to each other. Therefore, at the last iterations, the corresponding point pairs are not corrected. This means that the regression quality is the same as if the projective correspondence approach would not have been performed. Therefore, the additional corresponding point correction stage only reduces the number of ICP-iteration and speeds-up the process without changing the regression result.

4.2.8 3D Temporal Corners to 3D Model Registration to Handle Rotations

As already mentioned in section 2.3.2 on major limitation of fitting a 3D model into a 3D volume lies in gathering rotational movements due to the cylindrical symmetry of limbs. This also affects the determination of the pelvic pose which is of major interest for gait pa-

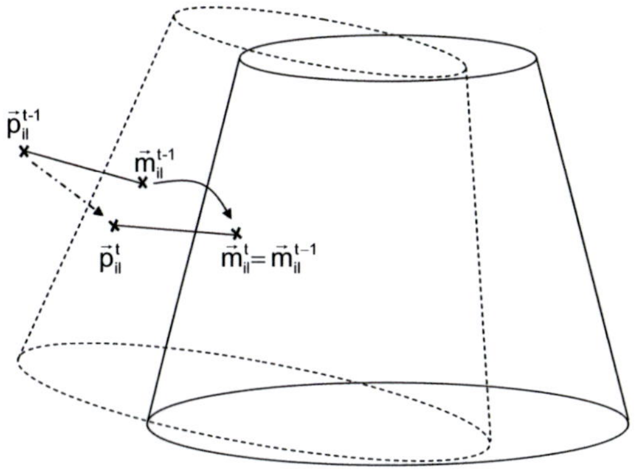

(a)

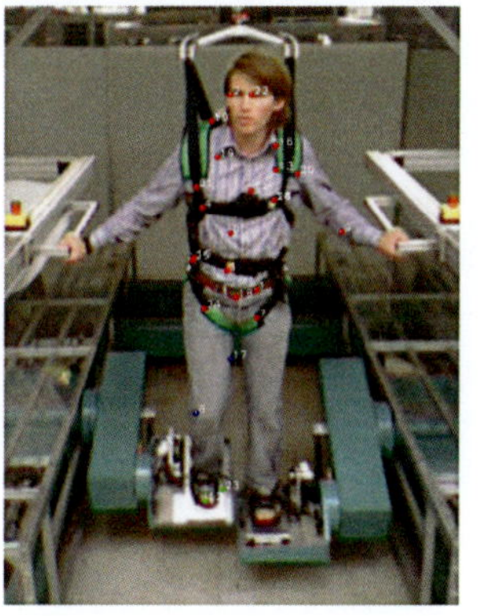

(b)

Figure 4.28: (a) visualizes the concept of the temporally tracked corners to overcome the *aperture problem* of the ICP-algorithm and track rotation. The corners are projected onto the model for further frames such that $\vec{m}_i^{t-1} = \vec{m}_i^t$. (b) An example of a set of corners marked as colored points.

rameter determination. The effect is closely related to the *aperture problem*[1] that is known from *stereo vision* or *optical flow* computation.

To overcome this *aperture problem* an approach is taken that determines an arbitrary set of unique corners c_i in 2D and tracks them over the previous three frames $\{t, t-1, t-2\}$ retrospectively. The main idea behind this is to determine a set of corresponding points $\mathcal{CP}_i$ that rely on unique correspondences. This is done by considering the previous projections of the unique corners onto the model. These globally tracked point correspondences effectuate the obviation of the *aperture problem* and yield a set of corresponding points $\mathcal{CP}_i$ that is not suffering from the *aperture problem.*

Tracking over three frames figured out to be a reasonable number of frames to get a sufficient amount of corners and to guarantee their consistency, i. e. their validity. Thereby, the validity of the corners is verified by incorporating the temporal consistency of the corner motion between frames in 3D. Corners which not resist this verification criterion are discarded.

The corners are determined by the *Speeded Up Robust Features* (SURF) operator [5] which basically is an accelerated version of the *Scale-Invariant Feature Transform* (SIFT) [61] by using a less complex mean filtering instead of a Gaussian filtering. But also the basic corner detector of *Shi* and *Tomasi* [96] provides a reasonable number of corners. The fig-

[1] The *aperture problem* describes the correspondence problem when only a locally limited field-of-view is considered for correspondence analysis. The locally limited field-of-view results in ambiguities in the correspondences. For example in stereo vision a homogeneously single-colored area does not allow for correspondence determination unless unique patterns such as textures get into the field-of-view. The correspondences of the remaining area can then be inferred from these unique correspondences.

ure 4.28(b) shows an example of a set of corners that are arbitrarily distributed over the body.
The 2D corners $\vec{c}_i = [x, y]^T$ are projected into 3D to $\vec{p}_{il} = [X, Y, Z]^T$ in the local body segment coordinates. Here, the index l labels points to be in the local limb 3D coordinate system. These 3D points are added to the point cloud $\mathcal{P}$ mentioned in the previous section 4.2.7 and used for the ICP based model fitting. But this time the corresponding point of $\vec{p}_{il}^t$ on the model $\vec{m}_{il}^t$ of the current frame at time step t is determined by taking the previous correspondence $\vec{m}_{il}^{t-1}$ since the tracked corners $\vec{c}_i$ keep their position on the model over frames. This can be expressed by:

$$\mathcal{CP}_{il}^t = \{\vec{p}_{il}^t, \vec{m}_{il}^t\} = \{\vec{p}_{il}^t, \vec{m}_{il}^{t-1}\} = \{\vec{p}_{il}^t, \vec{m}_{il}^{t-2}\} \tag{4.24}$$

Noise and the limitation of the model to express the reality is faced by taking the averaged previous correspondences $\vec{m}_{il}^{t-1}$ and $\vec{m}_{il}^{t-2}$ instead of the theoretical assumption from equation 4.24. Thereby, an increase of robustness is achieved. With this the equation 4.24 is rewritten to:

$$\mathcal{CP}_{il}^t = \{\vec{p}_{il}^t, \vec{m}_{il}^t\} = \{\vec{p}_{il}^t, \overline{(\vec{m}_{il}^{t-1}, \vec{m}_{il}^{t-2})}\} \tag{4.25}$$

The variation of the previous correspondences $\vec{m}_{il}^{t-1}$ and $\vec{m}_{il}^{t-2}$ define a measure of confidence for $\vec{m}_{il}^t$. If $\vec{m}_{il}^{t-1}$ and $\vec{m}_{il}^{t-2}$ vary excessively, $\vec{m}_{il}^t$ is discarded and not considered for further ICP processing.
Figure 4.28(a) illustrates this relation for a truncated cone which has moved between two subsequent time steps $(t, t-1)$. $\vec{p}_{il}^{t-1}$ is generated by projecting the corner c_i^{t-1} into 3D. Its corresponding point on the model $\vec{m}_{il}^{t-1}$ is determined by the closest point computation explained in the previous section 4.2.7.1 and should keep its local position on the model regardless of the motion that is tracked by the corner.
The corresponding point pair $\mathcal{CP}_i^t = \{\vec{p}_i^t, \vec{m}_i^t\}$ determined with the described strategy are used for ICP computation and provide a solution to incorporate internal-external rotations in the ICP computation.

4.2.9 3D Body Part Tracking - Hand Tracking to Handle Sparse Data Regions

Due to the currently low resolution of the TOF depth camera and the noise of the depth data it happens that the depth data of small body parts such as the hands, especially when moving, are sometimes segmented inaccurately. This makes it difficult to determine the corresponding point pairs $\mathcal{CP}_i^t = \{\vec{p}_i^t, \vec{m}_i^t\}$ for these body parts and, therefore, to track the hands correctly on the base of the reconstructed 3D data. This issue is displayed in figure 4.29.

To overcome this problem, the hands are tracked separately by a bottom-up approach in 2D which should feature fast processing. Since previous hand positions are present for this case and are used for initialization.

There are different tracking algorithms that can be separated into stochastic and deterministic ones. The search strategy differs such that the first one is stochastic and model-driven while the latter is deterministic and data-driven. A representative of the first group is the condensation algorithm introduced in computer vision by [42] (also particle, bootstrap or Sequential Monte Carlo filter) which is based on Monte Carlo integration methods. These methods perform a random search which is guided by a stochastic model to obtain an estimate of the posterior distribution that describes the object's configuration, here, the position of the hand. Thereby, multiple hypotheses are maintained simultaneously and a stochastic model is used to predict the position of the hand. The multiple hypotheses enable the method to recover from failure or temporary distraction and handle cluttered data. However, the maintainence of the hypotheses results in high computational costs for which reason such stochastic methods are not first choice for real time systems. A representative of the latter group is the mean shift algorithm introduced by

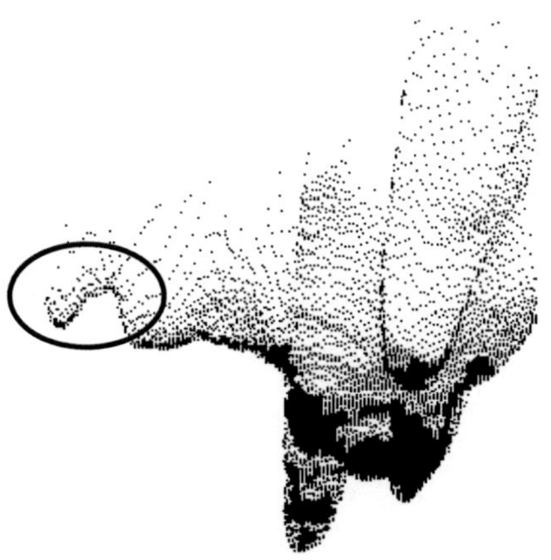

Figure 4.29: The figure shows a 3D point cloud $\mathcal{P}$ representing a human from bird eye's view where at the lower part of the point cloud the knees can be identified. The figure illustrates the problem of sparse data, here, appearing for the right hand. The foreground segmentation sometimes underperforms for small objects, like the hands. The blue ellipse encircles the apparently incorrect data of the right hand.

[30] and brought to computer vision by [13] and extended by [22] [21]. These methods localize an object based on a minimization of a cost function. It was demonstrated that this algorithm performs robustly in real-time. Additionally, this algorithm is able to cope with the variety of the appearances of the hand with its high number of DOF. An extension of the mean shift algorithm is the camshift (continuous adaptive mean shift), which itself adapts the size of the search window. For the considered purpose this self adaption is not necessary because the hands mostly stay within a certain range.
Therefore, in this thesis the latter category of approaches is chosen. In the following the mean shift algorithm and its adaption to depth data is explained similar to the proposal of [8] with a further adaption to increase depth dynamics.
The objective of the mean shift algorithm is to determine the position $\vec{x}_h^t$ in the current frame (time step t) for which a target candidate model $\hat{p}(\vec{x}^t)$ is as similar as possible in comparison to the to be tracked target model $\hat{q}$. The target $\hat{q}$ and the target candidate $\hat{p}(\vec{x}^t)$ are represented by its probability density function (PDF) in a chosen feature space which is usually given by the position in the image and the the color channels. For real-time reasons the PDF is represented in a discrete manner, i. e., a histogram with a fix number of D-bins is used. The similarity between the target $\hat{q}$ and the target candidate $\hat{p}(\vec{x}^t)$ is determined by applying a distance metric so that the minimization of the distance metric defines the most probable position of the hand $\vec{x}_h^t$ in the current frame. It is assumed that the tracked object moves slowly between successive frames and stays within a certain distance range. This assumption is required to set the starting position for the distance minimization to the hand position of the previous frame tracking result $\vec{x}_h^{t-1}$.
In contrast to most other works that use only the three channels of a color image, here, the depth channel is considered additionally. Therefore, four channels (L*, a*, b*, depth) and the position (x,y) in the image are used with $D = 16$ bins each. Since a distance measure is applied, the *CIE L*a*b** color space is used. The first three channels correspond to the *CIE L*a*b** channels. The 4th channel corresponds to the *depth data*. As dimension D of the histograms 16 yielded reasonable results in terms of accuracy and processing speed. This already results in 65536 possible combinations of the four channels. Doubling D would result in a multiplication by 16 of the possibilities of combinations and would rise the computational load significantly.
The target is represented by:

$$\hat{q} = (\hat{q}_1, \ldots, \hat{q}_d, \ldots, \hat{q}_D) \quad \text{with} \quad \sum_{d=1}^{D} \hat{q}_d = 1 \tag{4.26}$$

The target candidate is dependent of the position $\vec{x}^t$:

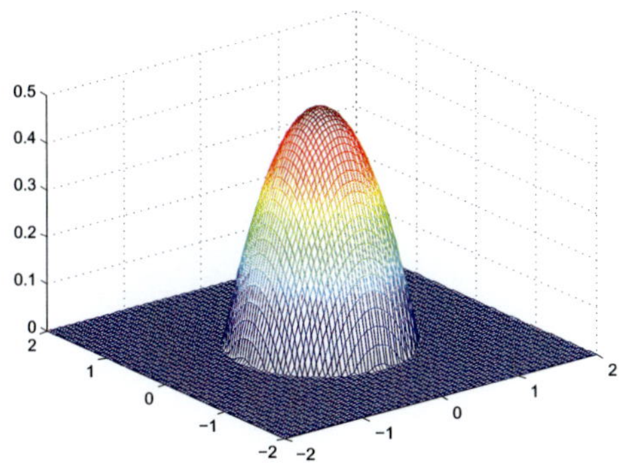

Figure 4.30: Used *Epanechnikov* kernel.

$$\hat{p}(\vec{x}^t) = (\hat{p}_1(\vec{x}^t), \ldots, \hat{p}_d(\vec{x}^t), \ldots, \hat{p}_D(\vec{x}^t)) \quad \text{with} \quad \sum_{d=1}^{D} \hat{p}_d = 1 \tag{4.27}$$

The similarity function between the two discrete PDF's $\hat{q}$ and $\hat{p}(\vec{x}^t)$ is denoted by:

$$\hat{\rho}(\vec{x}^t) \equiv \hat{\rho}[\hat{p}(\vec{x}^t), \hat{q}] \tag{4.28}$$

The function $\hat{\rho}(\vec{x}^t)$ represents the likelihood and its local maxima correspond to the target candidates $\hat{p}(\vec{x}^t)$ that are similar to the target $\hat{q}$. An optimization for this step is to regularize $\hat{\rho}(\vec{x}^t)$ by masking the objects with an isotropic [2] kernel in the spatial domain and estimate the PDF just within this kernel's weighted local area. Then, the function $\hat{\rho}(\vec{x}^t)$ becomes a smooth function because the kernel weights are smooth in their spatial domains. A differentiable kernel profile results in a differentiable similarity function $\hat{\rho}(\vec{x}^t)$. This makes it possible to apply gradient based maxima localization procedures. Therefore, various kernel profiles are suitable. In this work the *Epanechnikov*-kernel is used because it minimizes the *approximated mean integrated squared error* (AMISE) and, therefore, yields the best PDF estimation [94]. To support varying region sizes for the candidate target and the target, the considered regions are normalized to the unit circle with window size $wsz = 1$. The *Epanechnikov*-kernel is defined by:

$$K_E(x) = \begin{cases} \frac{1}{2} c_D^{-1}(D+2)(1 - ||x||^2), & ||x|| < 1 \\ 0, & \text{else} \end{cases} \tag{4.29}$$

[2]independent of spatial direction

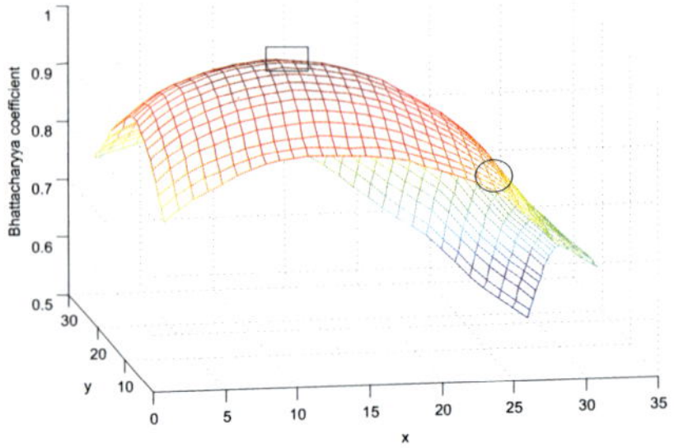

(a)

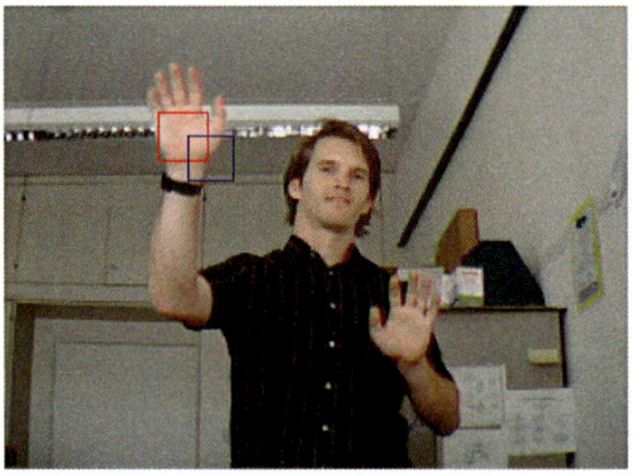

(b)

Figure 4.31: Example for the mean shift tracking based on the four channels L^*, a^*, b^* and *depth data*. (a) *Bhattacharyya*-coefficient estimate for the spatial coordinates (x, y). Starting from the circle (starting position $\vec{x}^t$) the kernel moves towards the square (target position $\vec{x}^t_h$). (b) corresponding color image with its starting position (blue square) and the target position (red square).

For the mean shift algorithm a metric is needed, which is able to compare the two histograms $\hat{q}$ and $\hat{p}(\vec{x}^t)$. There are different approaches for histogram comparison. The *Bhattacharyya*-coefficient is chosen as similarity function, because it performed well, but other metrics also work.

The *Bhattacharyya*-coefficient in the general exact form becomes a sum over the D-bins of the histograms for the discrete estimate:

$$\rho(\vec{x}^t) \equiv \rho[p(\vec{x}^t), q] = \int \sqrt{p_z(\vec{x}^t) q_z} dz \overset{\text{discrete estimate}}{\approx} \sum_{u=1}^{D} \sqrt{\hat{p}_u(\vec{x}^t)\hat{q}_u} \tag{4.30}$$

With the *Bhattacharyya*-coefficient a distance measure $d(\hat{p}(y), \hat{q})$ is constructed, which is used to finally determine the similarity between the two histograms, i. e., $\hat{q}$ and $\hat{p}(\vec{x}^t)$.

$$d(\hat{p}(y), \hat{q}) = \sqrt{1 - \rho[\hat{p}(y), \hat{q}]} \tag{4.31}$$

The updated position of the hand $\vec{x}^t_h$ is defined by the maximum of the *Bhattacharyya*-coefficient or the minimum of the distance measure $d(\hat{p}(y), \hat{q})$:

$$\vec{x}^t_h = \underset{\vec{x}^t}{\operatorname{argmin}} d(\hat{p}(\vec{x}^t), \hat{q}) = \underset{\vec{x}^t}{\operatorname{argmax}} \rho(\hat{p}(\vec{x}^t), \hat{q}) \tag{4.32}$$

A comprehensive description of the method is given by [21] and [22]. An example showing the density and the start and end position is given in figure 4.31.

An impression of the performance of the hand tracking algorithm is shown in figure 4.32. The figure shows some images of a test sequence. The red square marks the position of the tracked hands. The method tracks the hands robustly at a theoretical frame rate of $150 fps$ and this in spite of the many skin areas, like the face, the arms and the other hand. Short-term occlusion can even be compensated as shown in the bottom row of figure 4.32. Worth mentioning here, is the tracker does not loose track of the hand with the face as skin area in the background and the other hand in the front while both hands are moving. A previous recognition of the hands is not necessary because the hand positions of the tracking algorithm are initialized for each frame by the tracking results of the previous frame.

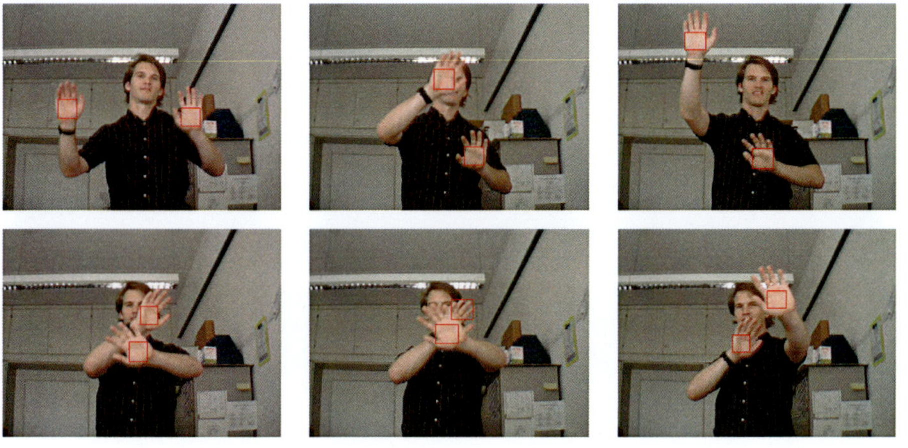

Figure 4.32: These images demonstrate the performance of the tracking. The tracked hands are marked with a red square. The method tracks the hands robustly at a theoretical frame rate of 150 *fps* and this in spite of the many similar skin areas, like the face, the arms and the other hand. Short-term occlusion can even be compensated as shown in the bottom row. The tracker does not loose track of the right hand although the face as skin area is the background and the other hand is in the front while both hands are moving.

5 Realization of the Demonstrator for Depth Data based Gait Parameter Determination

In this chapter the realization of the demonstrator for depth data based gait parameter determination and the generation of reference data is described.

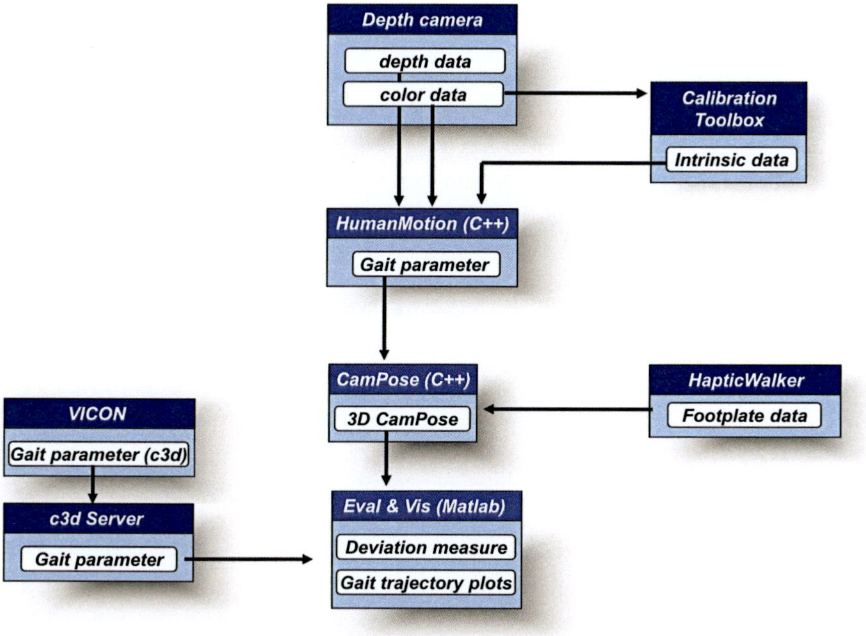

Figure 5.1: Interacting components of the realized system *HumanMotion* for the depth based determination of gait parameter trajectories. The boxes colored in light blue are the ones realized within this thesis, while the dark blue boxes are existing components, like software-libraries.

5.1 The Components of the Demonstrator

In this section, the individual components of the demonstrator and their interaction are briefly presented.
The demonstrator contains the realized components from section 4.1 and 4.2 for data acquisition, data processing / enhancement and posture synthesis. It consists of a TOF depth range imaging camera, of miscellaneous software libraries and tools as well of the developed software. Figure 5.1 displays the components and their interaction. Each component is illustrated by a box. The upper dark blue box denotes the component name. The white boxes inside the light blue boxes denote the results of the respective component which form the input for the component the arrow is pointing at. The blue boxes refer to the components realized in this work which might integrate extern components, such as software libraries, e. g., *OpenCV 2.0*[1] , while the dark blue boxes are whole systems, such as the marker based motion capturing system *Vicon*®[2]. In the following the components are described.
Two depth imaging cameras were investigated within this thesis. It was started with the *PMD [vision] 19k*[3] with a lateral resolution of 160 × 120 and switched over to the *3DVSystems ZCam*[4] with 320 × 240. The *PMD [vision] 19k* captures at 15 fps whereas the ZCam provides a frame rate of 30 fps. The opening angles are 40° for the PMD and 60° diagonal for the ZCam. The ranges of the two cameras lie between 0 – 7.5 m for the PMD [vision] 19k and between 0 – 3.5 m for ZCam. The *PMD [vision] 19k* shows an distance offset mean of 215 mm with a standard deviation of 41 mm due to the wiggling effect. The ZCam possesses a mean distance error of 153 mm with a standard deviation of 43 mm when applying for wide range. The *HapticWalker* forms the demonstrator scenario. It provides the positions of the foot plates. The *Calibration Toolbox*[5] is an open source toolbox implemented in *Matlab*[6]. It features functions for the determination of the intrinsic parameters of 2D cameras. For this calibration process a checker board is used. The calibration needed to be carried out only once for each depth range imaging camera to compensate for the lateral distortions and to rate the geometric projection error induced by this distortion to the depth data (see section 4.1.1 / 4.1.2). The intrinsic parameters are imported to *HumanMotion* through file-'read-in' as XML-format[7]. The software *CamPose* is developed to spatially synchronize the depth camera with the *Vicon*® marker based sys-

[1] http://sourceforge.net/projects/opencvlibrary/
[2] http://www.vicon.com/
[3] http://www.pmdtec.com/
[4] http://www.3dvsystems.com
[5] http://www.vision.caltech.edu/bouguetj/calib_doc/
[6] http://www.mathworks.de/
[7] http://www.w3.org/XML/

tem and the *HapticWalker* in an accurate and comfortable way. This is needed to provide a common coordinate system for reference and sample data. The transformation between these systems is computed from the calibration object of the marker based system that is used to define its origin. In figure 5.5(b) (page 99) the calibration object is displayed which will be further referred to as *L-Frame*. The software is explained in detail in section 5.3.4. *CamPose* is implemented in C++. The software *HumanMotion* is the main software that determines the joint angle trajectories on the base of the captured depth data. A comprehensive framework for data management, modeling, tracking and visualization is given by the software Voodoo[8] which was extended in this work [49]. A variety of additional software libraries, packages and programs is used. The software library *OpenCV 2.0* is used for image processing tasks [12]. But since *OpenCV 2.0* still just focuses on 2D image processing, several methods needed to be implemented for proper functionality. An extension of *OpenCV 2.0* is given by the library *OpenCVx*[9] which features additional methods and interfaces to, e. g., *Matlab* that are not yet integrated to *OpenCV 2.0*. The library *CXImage*[10] supplies required image format load functions not provided by *OpenCV 2.0*.The PMD and the ZCam API provide access to the depth range imaging cameras. For *Graphical User Interface* (GUI) the software[8] uses the window library *Qt*[11] and for 3D data and graphics rendering the *Coin3D*[12] as an *OpenGL*[13] based rendering library. It is basically an *SGI Open Inventor Clone* [14]. To integrate *Coin3D*'s 3D visualization in *Qt* the library *SoQt*[15] is used. Additional functionality in terms of, e. g., threading, string processing and data containers is given by the library *Boost C++ libraries*[16]. The software *HumanMotion* is implemented in C++. Its design features different software-design concepts, such as the *visitor* design pattern. The reference data was captured with the marker based *Vicon*® motion capturing system. The reference data is spatially synchronized with the depth data and, therefore, with the gait parameter trajectories which are provided by the software *HumanMotion*. The data is prepared for comparison with the *C3D server*[17] which basically is a Software Development Kit (SDK) providing access to the `c3d`-data format the *Vicon*® motion capture system uses to handle the captured marker's positions and joint angle traces. The comparison and visualization of the reference data with the gait traces data retrieved from *HumanMotion* is carried out within a developed software *Eval & Vis* that is implemented under *Matlab*. Additionally, within *Eval & Vis* some common

[8]http://sourceforge.net/projects/voodootracking/
[9]http://code.google.com/p/opencvx/
[10]http://www.codeproject.com/KB/graphics/cximage.aspx
[11]http://qt.nokia.com/
[12]http://www.coin3d.org/
[13]http://www.opengl.org/
[14]http://oss.sgi.com/projects/inventor/
[15]http://doc.coin3d.org/SoQt/
[16]http://www.boost.org/
[17]http://www.c3d.org/c3dapps.html

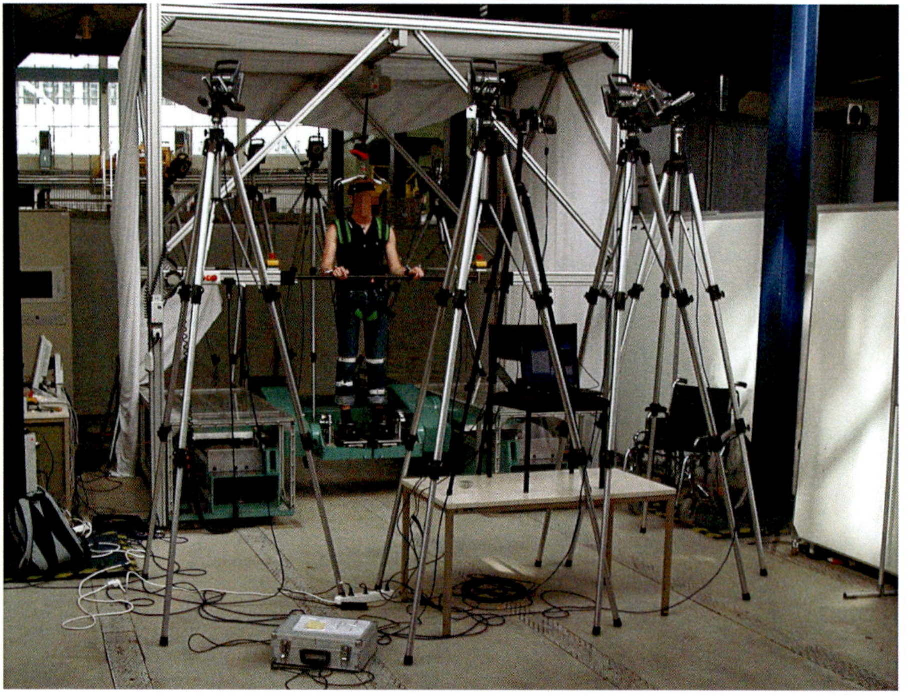

Figure 5.2: The system evaluation scene with a marker equipped person in the gait rehabilitation robot *HapticWalker*, the markerbased *Vicon*®-Motion Capture System with its 8 cameras and the used range imaging camera *3DVSystems ZCam*.

preprocessing methods for the gait trajectory data are implemented to perform filtering such as Kalman or Gaussian filtering.

5.2 Data Acquisition Scene and Demonstrator Scenario

Figure 5.2 gives an impression of the scene for reference data acquisition. A person which was equipped with markers in accordance with *Plug-In-Gait* marker set [24] was placed in the *HapticWalker*. The *Plug-In-Gait* marker set is described in section 5.3.2. These markers are captured and tracked by the 8 cameras of the used *Vicon*® 3D motion capture system. The range imaging camera *3DVSystems ZCam* is placed in front of the person in a height of 2.2m with an inclination angle of 30°. For easy and accurate spatial synchronization of the *Vicon*®-Motion Capture System and the *3DVSystems ZCam* a software *CamPose* was realized that determines the transformation between both systems on the base of the calibration object shown in figure 5.5(b). *CamPose* is described in section 5.3.4.

5.3 Reference Data Generation

The evaluation of the realized system to determine gait parameters is carried out by comparing the determined gait parameter trajectories with reference gait parameter trajectories. The reference gait parameter determination is described in this section.

5.3.1 *Vicon®* Markerbased Motion Capture System

For reference data generation a marker based 3D motion capture system of *Vicon®* is used. This system was partly financed through an university internal funding program to improve institutes' research facilities [52].

The system consists of eight cameras to compensate for marker occlusions. The cameras are of *T-Series* model type *T-10* equipped with a C-MOS sensor with a resolution of 1 mega-pixel and a maximum frame rate of 250 *Hz* for progressive scan mode. The illumination unit of each camera has 572 LED's of which 320 emit visible red light (623 nm) and 252 emit in near infrared light (780 nm). The LED's are arranged in a ring around the standard optics with a wide opening angle [101].

5.3.2 'Plug-In-Gait' Marker Set

The number and positioning of the markers is based on the type of motion being analyzed and the number of body segments needed to answer the research question. In this case the whole body needs to have markers attached to specific anatomical landmarks. The default whole body marker set used by the *Vicon®* system is the *'Plug-In Gait'* marker set. It is similar to the *Helen Hayes* marker set which is designed for clinical gait analysis.
The *Vicon® 'Plug-In Gait'* marker set basically is a self implementation of the *Conventional Gait Model* (CGM) introduced by Davis et. al. [24] which itself uses a modified *Helen Hayes* marker set of 16 markers on the hips and lower limbs. With the locations of these markers the joint centers are estimated on a frame-by-frame basis. Four markers placed around the pelvis are used to create a pelvic local coordinate system. The location of the pelvis joint center in this local coordinate system is estimated through a regression function. Figure 5.3(a) shows a person equipped with markers that were attached in accordance to the used *'Plug-In-Gait'* marker set. The Figure 5.3(b) shows a screen shot of the software

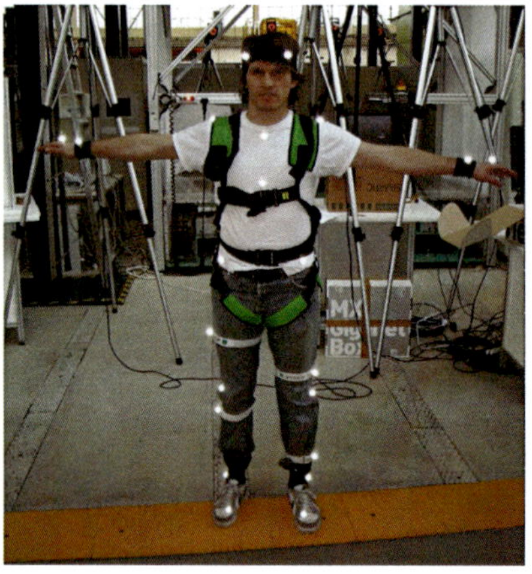

(a)

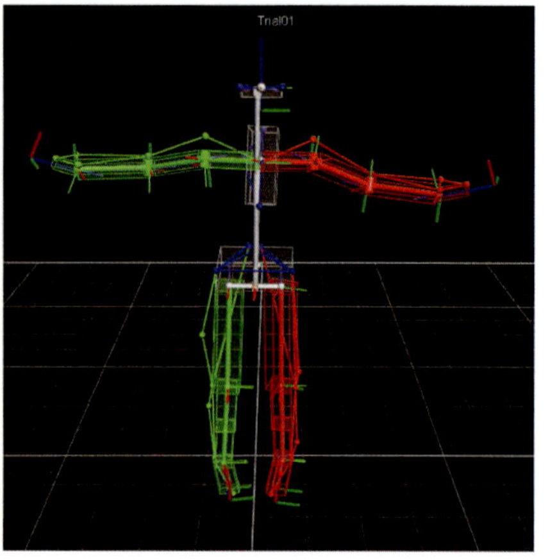

(b)

Figure 5.3: (a) A person with the attached marker set *'Plug-In-Gait'*. (b) A screen shot of the *Vicon®* *Nexus* software with the estimated joint positions along with a model skeleton of the person retrieved from the marker set.

Vicon® *Nexus* which computes joint positions and angles out of the tracked markers. In the screen shot the markers along with the estimated joint positions and an underlying skeleton is shown. A detailed description of the used *'Plug-In-Gait'* marker set is given in the appendix in section 8.1 for further information.

5.3.3 Side-by-Side Operation of *Vicon®*-System and Depth Camera.

For reference data generation the *Vicon®*-system and the depth camera are operated in side-by-side mode. Because both systems are based on IR-light, it needs to be guaranteed that the interaction, i. e., the influence of the *Vicon®* IR-strobe on the depth measurement not significant. The technical data of the IR-light emitting LED's used for the *Vicon®*-system and for the investigated depth cameras suggest that both systems can be operated side-by-side. The technical data of the TOF cameras and the marker based motion capture system are faced in the table 5.1.

In the technical data a statement about the sensitivity of the sensors with respect to IR-light bandwidth is not given. The *Vicon®*- system normally is used alone or with cameras that work on light within the visible spectrum. However, if this information would have been given, the question about the deviation induced by production variation would remain unanswered. Information about the bandwidth of the cameras is not available and cannot be measured due to lack of appropriate measurement equipment. Therefore, the

Feature	*Vicon®*-system	*3DVSystems ZCam*	*PMD [vision] 19k*
Wavelength [*nm*]	623 (320 units) / 780 (252 units)	830 (12 units)	870 (112 units)
Frame rate [*fps*]	120 (max.250)	30	max. 15

Table 5.1: Features of the *Vicon®*-system, *PMD [vision] 19k* and *3DVSystems ZCam*, [78], [99], [101].

side-by-side operation must be investigated directly.
Two experiments were carried out for this purpose:

1. The main principle of the first experiment is a comparative study. In this study a target is captured by the TOF camera. At one time the target is illuminated by the *Vicon® T10* camera strobe while at the other time not. The depth measurements of both scenarios are then compared. Thereby, different distances in 0.5m steps were investigated, i. e., 1.5m, 2m, 2.5m, 3m, 3.5m.

2. The second experiment aims to investigate the influences when the *Vicon® T10* camera strobe is aimed at the TOF camera. Thereby, the target is placed behind the *Vicon® T10* camera strobe and the distance is measured one time with the *Vicon® T10* camera strobe switched on and one time when it is switched off. These measured distances are compared. The setup for this is displayed in figure 5.4.

The frame rate of the *Vicon®*-system was chosen to be a multiple of the frame rates of the TOF cameras for synchronization (see table 5.1).

Since the frame rate of the *Vicon®*-system is a multiple of the depth camera's frame rate and, therefore, at least four strobes are captured, without any loss of generality it is valid to denoise the captured depth images by temporal averaging. Comparing the averaged depth images with and without illumination yielded a uniform behavior of the two depth

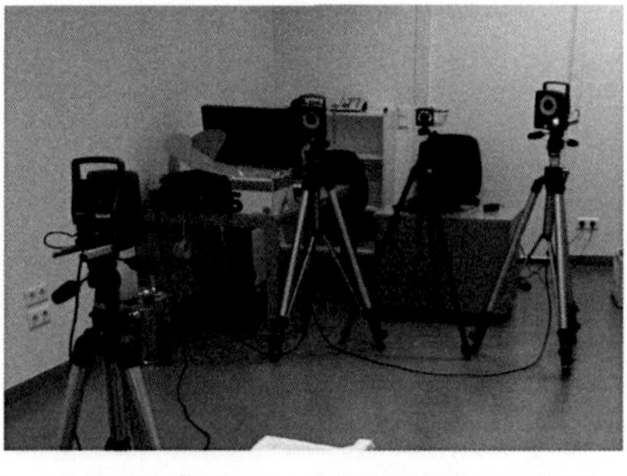

Figure 5.4: Setup to evaluate the influences of the IR-based *Vicon®*-system on the depth measurement of the IR-based TOF camera.

values per pixel throughout the distance range for both experiments. The results are listed in table 5.2. Because of the low deviations the influences between the *Vicon*®-system and the depth cameras are assumed to be insignificant and can be neglected.

	MEAN ERROR	STD. DEVIATION
Experiment 1 [cm]	0.36	0.74
Experiment 2 [cm]	-0.24	0.56

Table 5.2: This table lists the evaluation results of the two experiments to investigate the side-by-side influences of the *Vicon*®-system on the depth measurement of the TOF camera. The differences between depth values are small and, therefore, assumed to be insignificant.

5.3.4 Automated Sensor Origin Transformation

For the evaluation of the developed marker less optical motion capture system the reference data and the marker less captured gait traces data have to be fused on some abstraction level. Since these data are in 3D space, it is evident to fuse the data in 3D. For this purpose, the transformation between the marker based motion capturing system, providing the reference data, and the range imaging camera used for the marker less capture needs to be determined. This can be done by measuring the translation and the rotation which is hard to achieve accurately. Therefore, in order to avoid falling into the pitfall of measurement inaccuracy, the transformation is directly computed from the calibration object of the marker based system defining its origin. This calibration object that will be further referred to as *L-Frame* is described in an extra parenthesis on page 99 and is displayed in figure 5.5(b).

The main concept for the calculation of the transformation is to determine the markers' centers in a predefined order. In figure 5.5(b) this predefined order is illustrated by the L-Frame with the markers. The numbers adjacent to the single markers correspond to the order. Its relative spatial description is given in the parenthesis on page 99. The correspondences of the projections of the L-Frame's markers into the calibrated range image and the knowledge of the spatial structure of the L-Frame are used for computing the transformation. These correspondences between 2D and 3D are denoted by:

$$\vec{x}_i(x_i, y_i) \Leftrightarrow \vec{X}_i(X_i, Y_i, Z_i)\,|_{i=1,2,\ldots,5} \tag{5.1}$$

Here, $\vec{x}_i$ is a point in the image coordinate system and $\vec{X}_i$ is a point in the 3D coordinate system. The method is a two-stage method. The first stage can be described with the determination of the markers' centers with subpixel accuracy. The following section 5.3.4.1

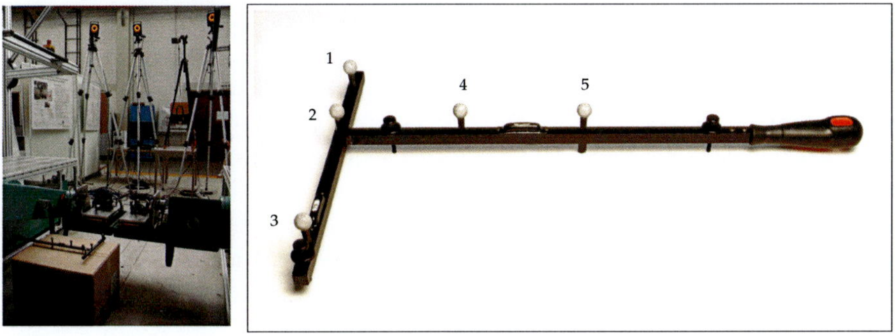

(a) (b)

Figure 5.5: (a) Scenario for automated transformation determination between TOF camera and *Vicon*®-system. The IR-cameras of the marker based system are mounted on the tripods as is the ToF range camera. The L-Frame is placed on the box to set the common origin for both systems and the *HapticWalker*. (b) shows the 5-marker L-Frame used for the automated transformation determination. The five markers of the calibration object displayed in white are numbered for reference.

is devoted to this stage. The second stage recovers the pose of the camera with respect to the L-Frame and is explained in section 5.3.4.2. Figure 5.5(a) displays the scenario the method is used for.

THE L-FRAME

The *L-Frame* is a calibration object that consists of two perpendicularly arranged straight bars with mounted reflective markers. The positions of the five markers on the two bars is shown in figure 5.5(b) along with the numbering for correspondence referencing. On each of the two bars there is one group of markers 1, 2, 3 on the one bar and markers 2, 4, 5 on the other bar. The marker number 2 is placed on the intersection of the two bars and defines the center of the coordinate system of the marker based system where the x-axis is along the markers 3, 2, 1 and the y-axis is along the markers 2, 4, 5. The distance between the markers 2↔4 and 4↔5 is 0.12m, the distance between markers 1↔ 2 is 0.08m and the distance between 2↔3 is 0.16m. Since the markers are omni reflecting and the range imaging camera is actively illuminating the scene, the markers can be segmented automatically in undefined environments. Just additional IR sources working in the same bandwidth have to be avoided. The marker based system's cameras do not influence the TOF camera.

5.3.4.1 Marker Center Determination

The determination of the correspondences between the positions of the markers in 3D $\vec{X}(X, Y, Z)$ and their projections in 2D $\vec{x}(x, y)$ forms an optimization problem which can be solved automatically. Since for the considered application this has to be done just one time no fully automated determination of the correspondences is needed. Therefore, the correspondences are determined by user interaction. That means that the regions of the markers of the *L-Frame* are marked separately for each marker in the camera image according to a predefined order. This order is illustrated by the numbers in the figure 5.5(b).

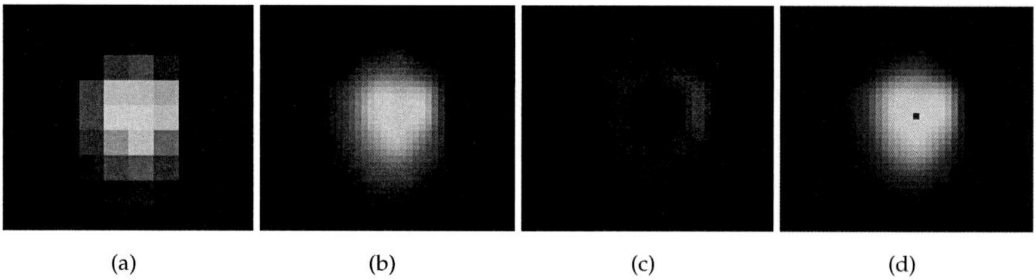

Figure 5.6: Different intermediate stages of the marker center determination. (a) shows the user selected ROI which is rescaled in (b) by factor four with a cubic interpolation. (c) shows the gradients and in (d) the found marker center is marked by a blue dot.

Based on these regions of interest (ROI) an algorithm for the computation of the markers' centers can be applied that assumes only one object to be in each ROI. Due to the low resolution of the camera a fitting of a circle into the data showed to be inaccurate. The figure 5.6 shows some intermediate stages of the marker center determination. The ROI's are of width N and height M. n_0 and m_0 are the top left coordinate of the extracted marker region. The gradient amplitudes both in x and y direction are computed using a 3×3 Sobel-Filter. Here, $D_x(x, y)$ is the intensity gradient in x-direction and $D_y(x, y)$ in y-direction. The error of the marker center computation is reduced by temporal smoothing of the considered images.

In both directions the gradient values are summed up if they cross a threshold th. This thresholding is implemented to suppress noise. With the *Kronecker-δ* and its boolean interpretation an intermediate value A_{cxm} for the x-direction is defined by:

$$A_{cxm} = \sum_{y=m_0}^{M} \underbrace{\sum_{y=m_0}^{M} \delta(|D_x(x, y)| > th_x)}_{\hat{A}_{cxm}} \tag{5.2}$$

The values of th_x and th_y are determined by scaling the maximum value of the gradient for each direction. A scaling factor of 50% figured out to be reasonable for both directions. The marker center $\vec{m}_c(x_{mc}, y_{mc})$ then results to:

$$\vec{m}_c(x_{mc}, y_{mc}) = (\frac{\sum_{x=n_0}^{N} \hat{A}_{cyn} \cdot x}{A_{cyn}}, \frac{\sum_{y=m_0}^{M} \hat{A}_{cxm} \cdot y}{A_{cxm}}) \tag{5.3}$$

The method is evaluated in a supervised way, i. e., the position of the markers' center determined by the method are compared to manually generated ground truth data. For this purpose, the images were scaled by factor 4. Thereby, a cubic interpolation was applied. The results are presented in the following table 5.3:

	MEAN ERROR	STD. DEVIATION
marker center accuracy [pxl]	0.2	0.33

Table 5.3: Accuracy of the automated marker's center determination.

5.3.4.2 Transformation Matrix Estimation

The pose of an object can be determined from single view using the method of [25]. This method is a combination of two algorithms, POS (Pose from Orthography and Scaling) and POSIT (POS with ITerations). POS computes the approximate pose and POSIT converges it to accurate pose measurements in a few iterations. The method provides the base for the transformation estimation.

The estimation of the transformation matrix is done by setting up an equation system on the base of 2D to 3D line and point correspondences and Direct Linear Transformation (DLT). Intrinsic camera and distortion parameters are assumed to be known beforehand. A detailed presentation of the mathematical background of the procedure is given in [28]. *OpenCV 2.0* provides appropriate methods for realization.

5.3.4.3 Evaluation of the Origin Transformation Estimation

The overall performance of the sensor origin transformation is evaluated in a supervised way. For this purpose, the transformations determined by the method are compared to ground truth reference data that is synthesized.

The evaluation setup is illustrated in figure 5.7. Here, $o - x_0y_0z_0$ represents the reference camera pose. The camera's pose is varied with respect to this reference pose. The varied camera pose is represented by $o' - x'y'z'$. $o_i - x_iy_iz_i$ is the L-Frame coordinate system. α is the total rotation of the camera around the $x - axis$.
The synthesized ground truth data are modeled with respect to the reference pose. For

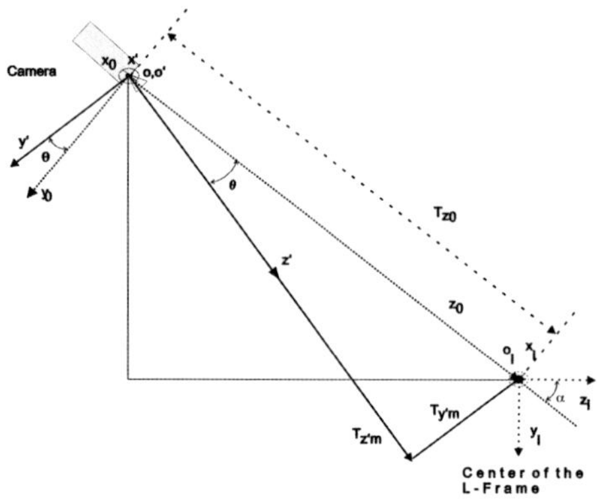

Figure 5.7: Camera coordinate system definitions and evaluation setup.

this purpose, T_{z0} is determined which is the distance between the camera center and center of the marker number 2 (see figure 5.5(b)) along the z direction when the camera is in reference pose. The distance T_{z0} is measured using a laser range finder which has a accuracy of $\pm 2mm$.

For evaluation the camera pose is varied with respect to the reference pose by varying the camera inclination angle θ_x. The evaluation process considers three values: T_z, T_y and θ_x. Especially T_z is considered since it is evidently the weakest point for single view pose estimation. Two models are used to synthesize the translational ground truth data $T_{z'm}$ and $T_{y'm}$. These values describe the translational distance between the centers of the camera and marker number 2 in z and y direction for rotations around $x-axis$ (see figure 5.7). These are the values which are compared with the computed values T_z and T_y of the realized method. In the ideal case they should be the same. The distance $T_{z'm}$ and $T_{y'm}$ are modeled by:

$$\begin{aligned} T_{z'm} &= T_{z0} \cdot cos(\theta_x) \\ T_{y'm} &= T_{z0} \cdot sin(\theta_x) \end{aligned} \tag{5.4}$$

The figure 5.8 displays the relation between the computed and the synthesized ground truth values of the translation vector for evaluation data set 1. It can be observed that the values of the estimated translation vector are very close when the angle θ_x is in positive direction. Here, the mean error in z direction is $-0.68\ cm$ and a standard deviation of $2.55\ cm$ The errors for another evaluation data set 2 are similar to the errors of evaluation data set 1. The mean error in z direction for the evaluation data is $0.50\ cm$ and a standard deviation of $3.08\ cm$. The peaks within the angles $-10.0 \geq \theta \geq -2.0$ for the evaluation data set 1 are due to the measurement inaccuracy.

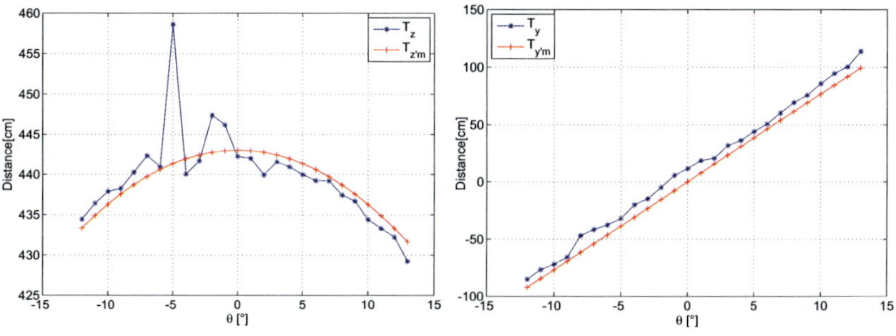

Figure 5.8: Evaluation data set 1: Modeled ground truth values of $T_{z'm}$ & $T_{y'm}$ and the values T_z & T_y that were computed with the realized method for rotations around the $x - axis$.

The evaluation of the rotational component around *x-axis* figured out to be 1.96° and 1.52° in standard deviation while assuming an unbiased error due to the unstable reference angle determination. To obtain the standard deviation with an unbiased error first a *multiple linear regression (MLR)* that uses least squares is applied. This is due to the measurement errors for reference setup as well as due to the alignment of the tripods rotation axis and the camera optic center which is hard to achieve.

The accuracy of the realized method to compute the transformation matrix on the base of 2D to 3D point correspondence is competent although showing inaccuracies. The error in the computation of the translation matrix is about $\pm 1cm$ and for the rotation matrix it's about $\pm 2°$.

Since only considering distances of less than $4m$ the subpixel determination of the centers of the projected markers in the image introduce a maximum error for T_y of only $0.2cm$ which can be determined by some basic trigonometry. T_z are affected less (see figure 5.7). Therefore, the realized method is competent for 3D data fusion.

As an overview, the results of the evaluation are presented in the following table 5.4:

	MEAN ERROR	STD. DEVIATION
T_z data set 1 [cm]	-0.68	2.55
T_z data set 2 [cm]	0.50	3.08
T_y data set 1 [cm]	-0.17	1.74
T_y data set 2 [cm]	0.91	2.23
θ_x data set 1 [°]	0.0	1.96°
θ_x data set 2 [°]	0.0	1.52°

Table 5.4: Overview of evaluation results of the accuracy of the automated origin transformation determination.

6 Evaluation

Within this chapter the evaluation of the described and realized system is presented and evaluated with respect to the objectives (see section 3).

Concerning the criteria related to *'Determination of the relevant gait parameters'* all relevant gait parameters are determined, except the ankle joint angle because it can be determined by considering the footplate angle of the *HapticWalker*. The different aspects of the criterion *'Accuracy'* are presented separately. Besides the overall accuracy of the gait parameter determination (section 6.2) the sensor accuracy is presented in section 6.1 because the TOF camera a relatively new sensor. The evaluation of the criterion *'Clinical Applicability'* is described in section 6.3.

6.1 Sensor Data Accuracy of TOF Range Imaging Cameras

Because the most significant error source is the error induced by different reflectivities of the targets, this section refers to results of reducing this error source.

In this thesis, two TOF camera models were investigated. At the beginning of this work the *PMD [vision] 19k* was used which was later on exchanged by the *3DVSystems ZCam* that shows a higher performance with respect to frame rate and resolution. Because the investigations about the data enhancement for the *PMD [vision] 19k* forms a valuable base for the investigations about the *3DVSystems ZCam*, the results achieved for this camera are also presented. The results are presented separately for both TOF cameras. First, the achieved results for the *PMD [vision] 19k* and then for the *3DVSystems ZCam* are evaluated.

6.1.1 Depth Data Enhancement Results for *PMD [vision] 19k*

The sensor accuracy is dependent on the achieved sensor data enhancement. Therefore, the achieved enhancement is determined. In order to determine the enhancement potential of the developed method in relation to state-of-the-art methods, the developed method and the state-of-the-art methods are applied on the same depth data. The achieved results are then compared.

For the evaluation of the realized depth data enhancement method a supervised evaluation technique is used. For this purpose a subset of samples of the amplitude range was used to build up the **L**ook-**U**p-**T**able (LUT) which is afterwards applied to the remaining amplitudes for correction. 5 samples of the amplitude range in every LUT of the third stage were selected to construct new LUT's. With these new LUT's the remaining data which was not used for LUT construction is corrected and compared with the nominal distance.

There are two experiments for both of the most related works. Within the first experiment the potential of the developed method is compared against the calibration method published by Kahlmann et. al. in [46] by applying both methods on the same data. The other experiment provides a comparison of the results of the proposed calibration with the one published by Lindner et. al. in [58].

Because the proposed calibration method extends the method of [46] by an additional third stage, the first experiment gives an impression of the potential of the third stage by comparing the potential with and without this third stage. The potential without the third stage is shown in figure 6.1(a) whereas the figure 6.1(b) shows the potential with

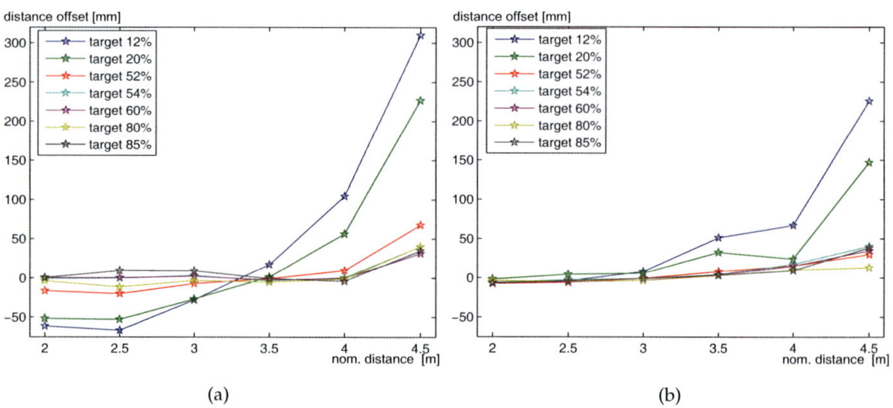

Figure 6.1: Both figures show the distance offset (i. e., the distance error) against its nominal distances (i. e., the real distance) for targets with different reflectivity (indicated by the amount of reflected light in %). (a) after the Look-up-table (LUT) based calibration of [46]. (b) after applying the proposed calibration. The distance error has been reduced and all targets present a more similar behavior regardless of their reflectivity.

applying the third stage. It can be seen that by applying the third stage the distance error is significantly reduced for targets regardless of their reflectivity. The underlying data of these plots are listed in the tables 6.1 and 6.2. Table 6.1 refers to figure 6.1(a) and table 6.2 to figure 6.1(b).

INT. TIME [ms]	DIST. [m]	DIST. ERROR [mm]		
		T_{20}	T_{52}	T_{80}
21.0	2.0	-51.7	-16.4	-3.9
30.0	2.5	-52.8	-20.0	-11.6
39.0	3.0	-26.9	-7.2	-3.3
27.0	3.5	7.1	-1.0	-5.4
42.0	4.0	56.3	9.6	-1.2
36.0	4.5	226.7	67.9	40.3

Table 6.1: Distance error in mm **without** applying the newly introduced third stage for different nominal distances in m and targets with different reflectance. The sub index represents the percentage of reflectance property of the target.

INT. TIME [ms]	DIST. [m]	DIST. ERROR [mm]		
		T_{20}	T_{52}	T_{80}
21.0	2.0	-1.6	-7.3	-3.6
30.0	2.5	4.4	-5.7	-4.5
39.0	3.0	5.9	-0.6	-3.4
27.0	3.5	38.5	7.1	-2.9
42.0	4.0	24.1	15.6	10.9
36.0	4.5	146.8	30.1	13.2

Table 6.2: Distance error in mm **after** applying the proposed calibration method for different nominal distances in m and targets with different reflectivities. A significant improvement in comparison to the most related method of Lindner et. al. [58] was achieved. The sub index represents the percentage of reflectance property of the target.

Table 6.3 shows the results of the second experiment. On the left side the results of Lindner et. al. from [58] for 1.7m and targets with a reflectivity of 20% and 80%. The sub index represents the percentage of reflectance property, the sub index A refers to the average. On the right side are shown the distance errors after applying the proposed calibration method for 2m and with targets with reflectivities of 20%, 52%, and 80% in a scale where 0% references a total absorber. In comparison with the method presented by

Lindner et. al. in [58], the proposed method performs better for the available comparable data. Additionally, our method covers a bigger range of distances.

DIST. ERROR [MM] from [58]			DIST. ERROR [MM] PROP. METHOD		
T_{20}	T_A	T_{80}	T_{20}	T_{52}	T_{80}
11.3	9.7	4.2	-1.6	-7.3	-3.6

Table 6.3: Distance error in mm **after** calibration with the proposed method at a distance of $2m$ in comparison with results of the most related work of Lindner et. al. from [58] at a distance of $1.7m$ for objects with different reflectivities. The sub index represents the percentage of reflectivity of the target, the sub index A refers to the average.

In this work the up to now unknown distance and integration time dependency over the behavior of the error against the amplitude has been described. Concretely, it has been observed that between $2m$ and approximately $3.5m$ the signed distance offset increases with the amplitude, whereas between $3.5m$ and $7m$ it decreases with the amplitude. In order to cope with this behavior, a three-stage calibration method has been proposed. The first two stages of the method handle the part of the distance and integration time errors which do not depend on the amount of incident light by applying LUT's first published in [46]. The third stage corrects the effect of the incident light on distance offset by taking into consideration the amplitude, the integration time and the pre-corrected measured distance.

A significant reduction of the distance error is achieved compared with existing calibrations. Compared with the calibration method proposed in [58], better results are achieved. Moreover, the proposed calibration method is applicable for a wider range of distances. The improvements are listed in the table 6.4.

	MEAN ERROR			STD. DEVIATION		
	T_{20}	T_{52}	T_{80}	T_{20}	T_{52}	T_{80}
uncorrected depth [mm]	70.25	20.35	10.95	78.98	24.25	14.80
corrected depth [mm]	36.88	11.07	6.43	55.69	10.50	4.45
IMPROVEMENT RATE	47.50%	45.62%	41.25%	69.97%	56.70%	29.48 %

Table 6.4: In this table a qualitative value of the depth data enhancement for the above sample is given. The high reduction of the std. deviation demonstrates a reduction of the dependency of the reflectivity onto the depth measure. The reduction of the mean error spreads over the whole band of reflectivities.

6.1.2 Depth Data Enhancement Results for *3DVSystems ZCam*

Because of the lack of related data enhancement methods for the *3DVSystems ZCam*, the enhancement potential of the developed method is determined by comparing the corrected data with the uncorrected data.

A comparative study of the uncorrected and the corrected depth data is shown in figure 6.2. It demonstrates the potential of the data correction. To provide a more comparative presentation a constant offset had not been applied which additionally needs to be applied for full correction. The figure clearly shows the reduction of the influence of the reflectivity of the targets being captured by incorporating a reflectivity estimation.

A more practical impression of the potential of the algorithm is shown in the figures 6.3 which displays one rgb-image (image 6.3(a)) and two depth data images of the same scene. The image 6.3(b) shows the uncorrected data whereas the image 6.3(c) shows the image after being corrected with the proposed method. The improvement of the depth data after correction can clearly be identified by a reduction of the distance offset variation on person's body. Note that the algorithm was applied after foreground segmentation so that background was not corrected.

The quantitative evaluation of the proposed method for depth data enhancement is given in table 6.5. Flat objects with different reflectivities were used to solely investigate the

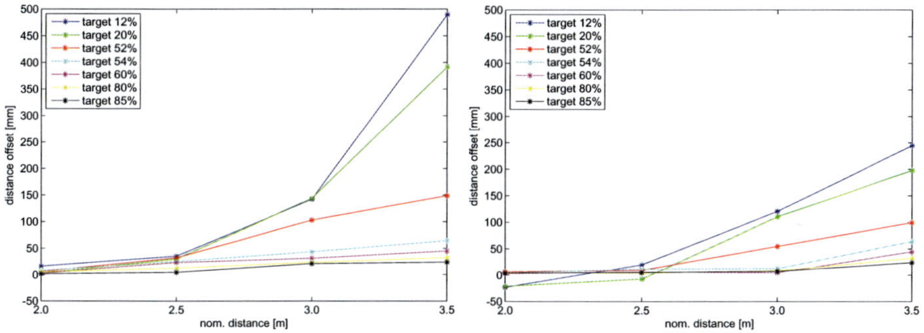

(a) (b)

Figure 6.2: Both figures show the distance offset (i. e., the distance error) against its nominal distances (i. e., the real distance) for targets with different reflectivity (indicated by the amount of reflected light in %). (a) **before** applying any depth data enhancement. (b) **after** applying the proposed calibration. The distance error has been reduced and all targets present a more similar behavior regardless of their reflectivity. Only targets with a low reflectivity show a significant error in terms of the objectives.

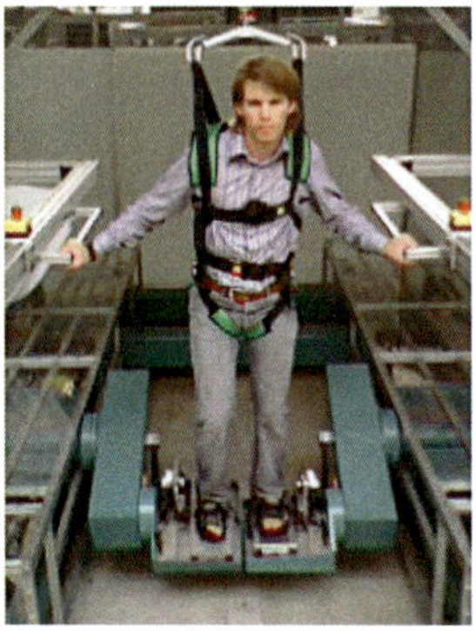

(a)

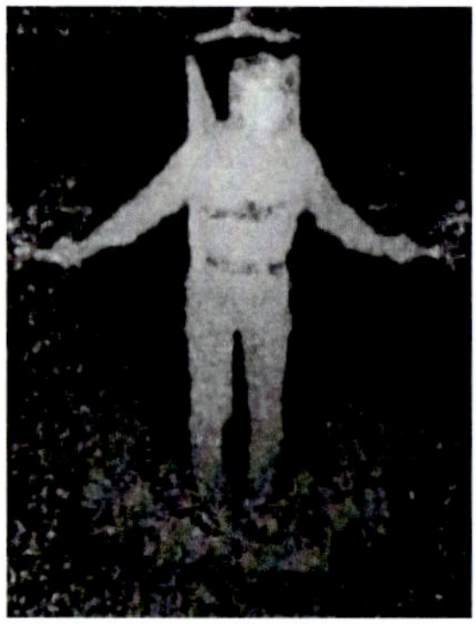

(b)

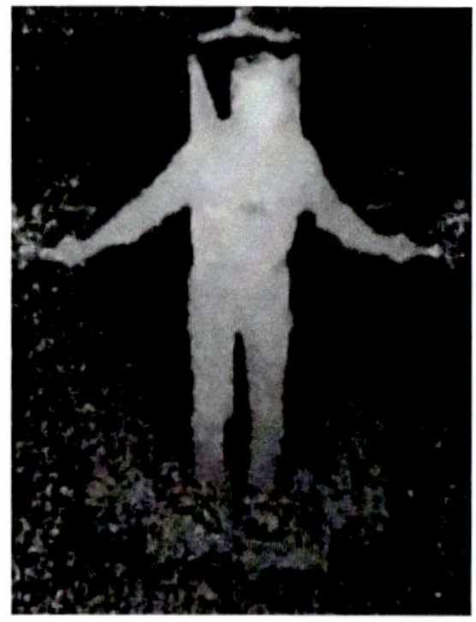

(c)

Figure 6.3: Illustration of the potential of the proposed algorithm. (a) shows the captured scene. The person as object of interest shows body areas with different reflectivities appearing as lighter and darker regions, e. g. the black belt with a low reflectance. These different regions result in a different distance error. This is supported by the depth data displayed in figure (b). Here, for instance the black belt can clearly be identified in the depth data. Figure (c) displays the depth data after being corrected with the proposed algorithm.

reflectivity issue. For this purpose a supervised evaluation was carried out that incorporates the depth values with and without the depth correction. As parameters for the evaluation the mean value and the standard deviation are used. Here, the mean value can be interpreted as a overall measure and the standard deviation as a measure how the proposed method is able to handle different objects' reflectivities. A reduction of the *mean error* and a reduction of the *standard deviation* is achieved with the developed method.

	MEAN ERROR			STD. DEVIATION		
	T_{20}	T_{52}	T_{80}	T_{20}	T_{52}	T_{80}
uncorrected depth [mm]	147.75	72.50	19	171.85	65.43	11.91
corrected depth [mm]	70.25	43.04	12.75	103.72	43.88	13.67
IMPROVEMENT RATE	52.45 %	40.69 %	32.89 %	39.65 %	32.93 %	14.73 %

Table 6.5: Mean and standard deviation of the depth data enhancement for selected reflectivities of the above sample.

6.1.3 Evaluation

PMD [vision] 19k

Evaluating the achieved results with respect to the objective shows that an accuracy of 0.01m is achieved within a range of 1.0m to 3.5m. However, this only applies to objects that have a reflectivity of at least 52%. Therefore, this model is not suited for objects with a reflectivity of less than 52%.

3DVSystems ZCam

Interpreting the achieved results with regard to the objective shows that an accuracy of 0.01m can be achieved within a range of 1.5m to 3.0m. Due the opening angle of the camera of 60° the movements of a person can be captured completely from a maximal distance of 3.0m. However, these results, as for the other camera, show that the model performs best for objects with a high reflectivity and is not suited for objects with a low reflectivity. A reflectivity of at least 54% is needed to provide data with an accuracy of 0.01m that corresponds to the objectives.

6.2 Gait Parameter Accuracy

In this section the gait parameter trajectories, which are determined with the realized system, are presented and their accuracy is evaluated in section 6.2.3.

The evaluation of the accuracy of the determined gait parameters is carried out by comparing them with reference gait parameters of the same scene that are acquired simultaneously. A markerbased *Vicon*®-system is used to capture the reference data (see section 5.3). The gait parameter accuracy is determined for the considered demonstrator scenario (HapticWalker) as described in section 5.2. The figure 6.4 shows a selection of sample 2D images captured with the TOF camera for gait parameter determination. The markers that are attached to the body for reference data generation appear as white spots.

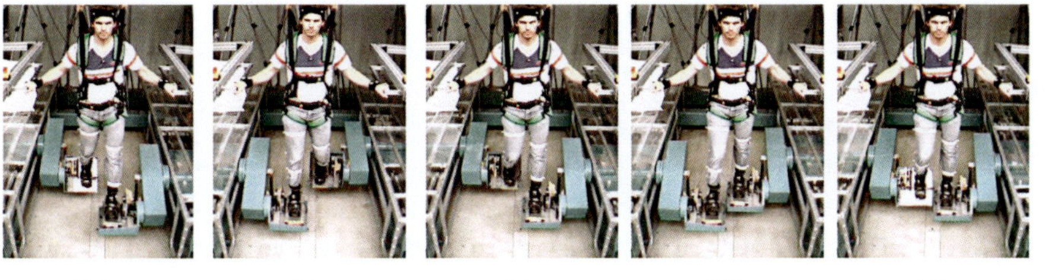

(a) (b) (c) (d) (e)

Figure 6.4: Sample images of an evaluation sequence.

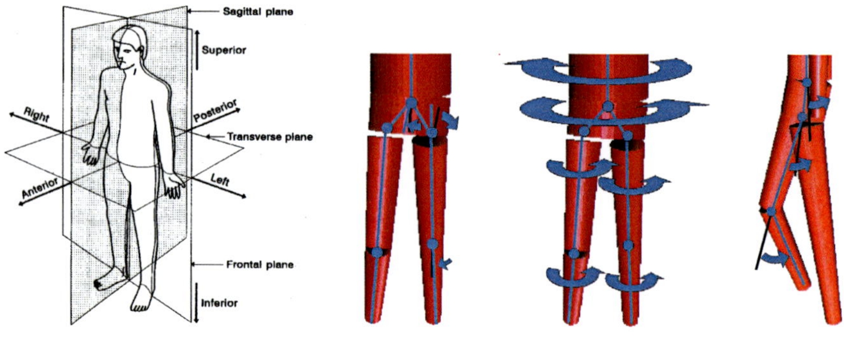

(a) (b) (c) (d)

Figure 6.5: Angles for the different considered joints (pelvis, hip and knee) and for the different planes (frontal, sagittal and transverse) (see (a) [105]). To depict the angles of the model a stick figure is super-imposed. The angles always relate to the parent limb whose orientation is depicted by the black lines. The arrows define the positive direction. Figure (b) shows the angles in the frontal plane, (c) in the transverse plane and (d) in the sagittal plane.

The gait parameters are represented by their temporal trajectories over a whole gait cycle. In order to be able to interpret these gait parameter trajectories, some definitions need to be known. For the interpretation of the joint angle trajectories, a definition of the joint angles is necessary. Figure 6.5 visualizes the angles for the three different planes, i. e., the frontal, the sagittal and the transverse plane (see figure 2.1). The joint angles are defined by the orientation of the neighboring two body segments. The angles always reference to the orientation of the parent limb according to the model hierarchy defined in section 4.2.4 (see figure 4.19(a)). The parent limb orientation is depicted in figure 6.5 by the black lines. The angles are given in positive direction.

The joint angle trajectories are plotted against the percentage of the gait cycle for the right leg starting with the *initial heel contact* (see section 2.2.1). This is the standard representation in gait analysis. The time for one gait cycle which is needed for this representation is calculated of the cadence[1] settings of the *HapticWalker*. To synchronize the reference trajectory and the trajectory that was measured with the developed system, the *initial heel contact* is used.

Additional to the joint angle trajectories, the movement of the pelvis is plotted. This enables the therapist to evaluate the symmetry of the weight takeover from one leg to the other.

Figure 6.6 is an example of gait parameter trajectory plots how they are presented in this work. The gait parameter plots always show the *mean* and the *standard deviation* over 10

[1] stride frequency [strides per minute]

gait cycle. Therefore, there are always three lines for one parameter trajectory with the positive and negative *standard deviation* wrapping the *mean*. The angles of the left side leg are plotted in 'green' and the angles of the right side are plotted in 'red'. The reference trajectory is plotted as a gray area which is defined by the trajectory's standard deviation. The joint angle trajectories are always presented by two figures which show the trajectory with different scales. In the left figure the angle trajectories are plotted with a range that is standardly used in gait analysis [88]. The right side figure shows the same plot, but with a different range so that details become more visible.

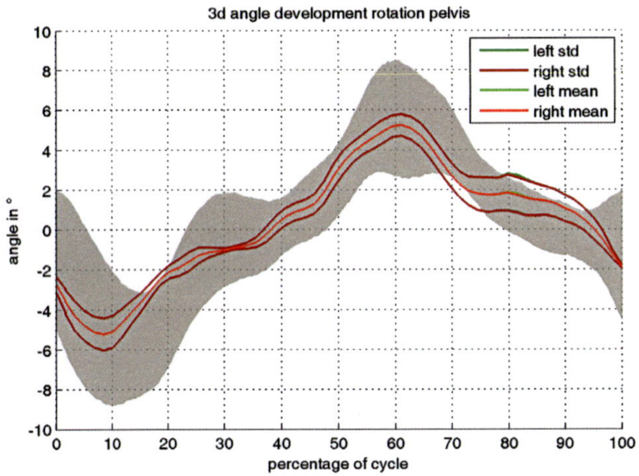

Figure 6.6: Example of the gait parameter trajectories presentation as it is used in this work.

6.2.1 Joint Angle Trajectories

Within this section the joint angle trajectories that are determined with the realized system are presented in the order: pelvis, hips and knees. A discussion about the achieved results follows in section 6.2.3. For each joint two of the captured evaluation sequences are presented.

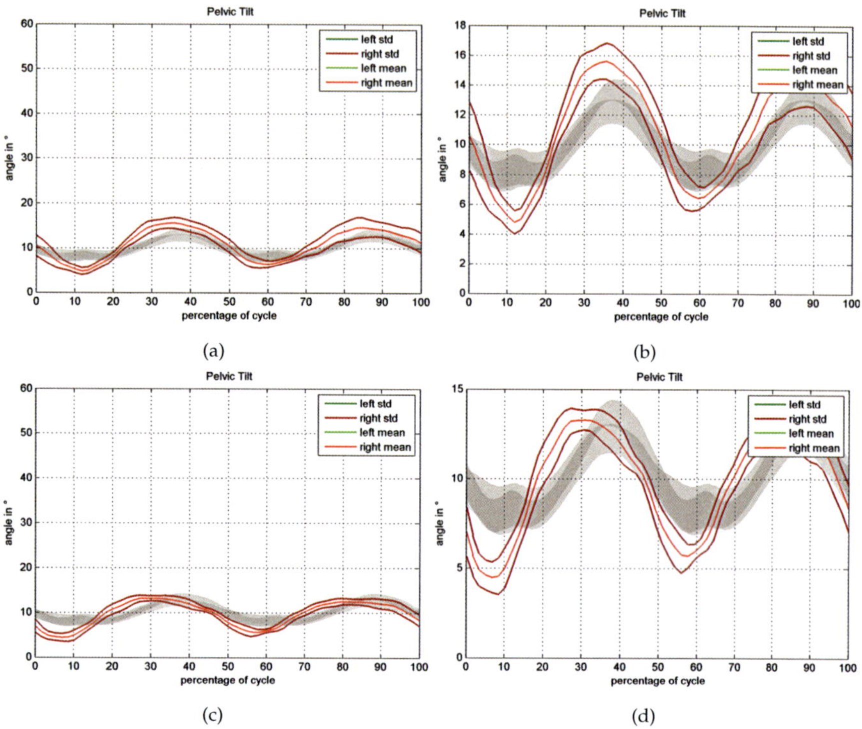

Figure 6.7: Trajectories of the rotational movements of the pelvis in the sagittal plane (pelvic tilt).

In figure 6.7 the rotational movements of the pelvis in the sagittal plane (pelvic tilt) are plotted. The figures (a) and (b) of the upper row belong to one sequence and the figures (c) and (d) of the bottom row belong to another sequence.

The figures show that the general trend of the determined trajectories equals the reference trajectories. Both trajectories have a sinusoidal characteristic with two maxima and two minima. Although the trend is the same, a slight phase shift of 5% of the gait cycle towards the beginning of the gait cycle can be noted. This phase shift can be explained by the relatively small visible surface of the pelvis and the camera's small resolution. Therefore, the pelvis is sampled by less 3D points than its neighboring body segments which have a bigger surface. Because these neighboring body segments are physiologically connected to the pelvis, the pelvis' movement is influenced by their movements. Especially the pelvis is prone to this effect because of its relatively small surface and the resulting fewer 3D points with which it is sampled.

The mean angle deviations between the determined and the reference trajectories are al-

ways less than 6°. Within this context it should be restated that this nearly matches the worst case angle mean squared error of 7° of a markerbased-system [56].
Another influence is given by the soft tissues, like the clothes which do not accurately represent the underlying pelvis. This is due to the folds of the trousers which are particularly big at the pelvis. The section 6.2.3 presents an experiment which reduces these different influences on the measurement to demonstrate the functionality.

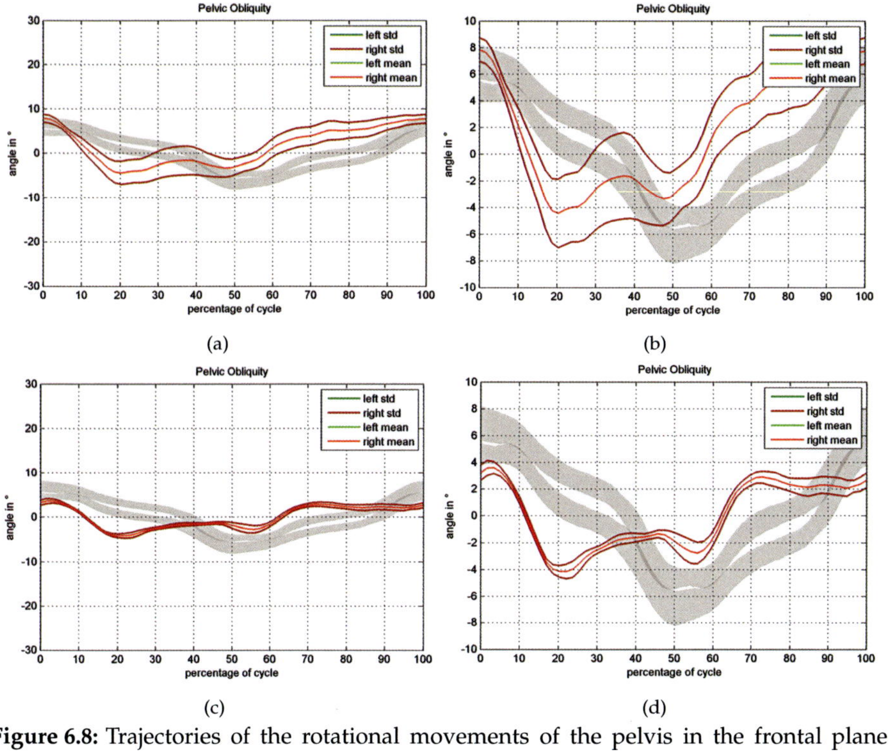

Figure 6.8: Trajectories of the rotational movements of the pelvis in the frontal plane (pelvic obliquity).

Figure 6.8 shows trajectories of the pelvic obliquity angle which is the rotational movement in the frontal plane (see figure 6.5(a)). The determined joint angles show a global minimum and a maximum at the beginning of the gait cycle which corresponds to the reference trajectories. From 5% to 20% of the gait cycle an increased downward slope of the plot in the single support phase can be noted. The upward slope is comparable to the reference trajectory slope but starts too early at 20%. Generally, the determined trajectory amplitude is slightly smaller than the amplitude of the reference trajectory. The angle deviations between reference and measured data are at maximum 7° which is slightly more than the worst case reference angle error [56]. As already mentioned, for a discussion about the causes for the deviations the reader is referred to the following section 6.2.3 which presents an experiment which reduces the different influences on the measurement and therefore allows for an assessment of the error causes.

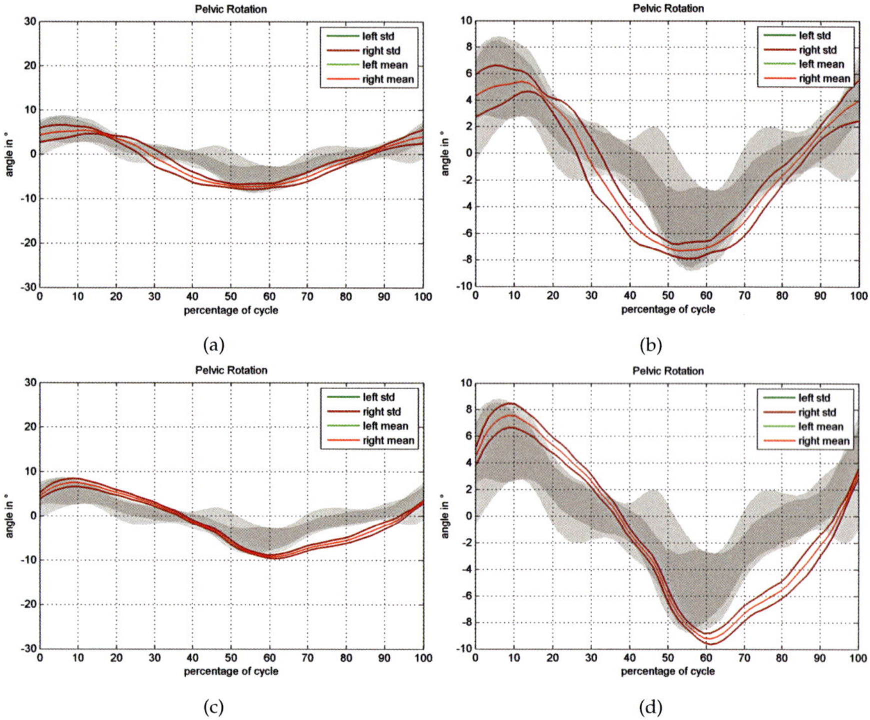

Figure 6.9: Trajectories of the pelvic rotational movements in the transverse plane (pelvic rotation).

Figure 6.9 shows the pelvic rotation angle trajectories. The trend of the joint angle trajectories equal the reference data trajectories for both sequences. The angle deviations between reference and measured data are at maximum 4°. This is especially worth mentioning, because the total absolute angular range of the obliquity is just 16°. The pelvic rotation is generally well captured with the realized system. This counts also for the symmetry of the gait, because the symmetry of the reference data equals to the symmetry of the measured angles. For a discussion about the causes for the deviations, the following section 6.2.3 presents an experiment which reduces the different influences on the measurement and therefore allows for a assessment of the error causes.

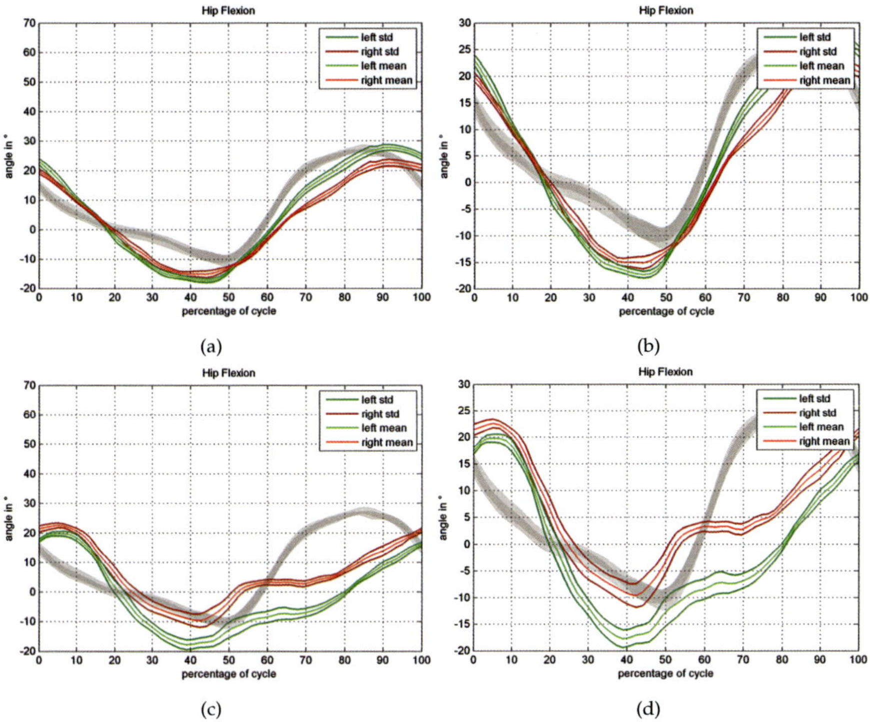

Figure 6.10: Trajectories of the angles of the hip flexion which is the angle between the thigh and the pelvis in the body's sagittal plane (see figure 6.5(a) and (d)).

Figure 6.10 shows the hip flexion which mainly effects the forwards/backwards movement of the leg (see figure 6.5(a) and (d)). Again, the overall trend of the reference trajectories is reflected by the determined hip flexion trajectory. Both joint angle trajectories show a minimum at 45-50% of the gait cycle. The range of the determined angles also equals to the range of the reference. Right before the minimum at 40% of the gait cycle a slight overrun can be noted. This inaccuracy results from inaccuracies of other joint angles during this phase of the gait cycle. This means that the increased hip flexion is due to an angle error at other joints which transfer to the hip joint. Especially, in this case the increased hip flexion can be put down to a decreased hip adduction. See the figure 6.11 for comparison. Just for the lower sequence in figure 6.10(d) a relatively low hip flexion during swing phase starting at 60 % of the gait cycle can be noted. In this case the slightly higher pelvic rotation is responsible for this, because the increased pelvic rotation causes the hip flexion to decrease.

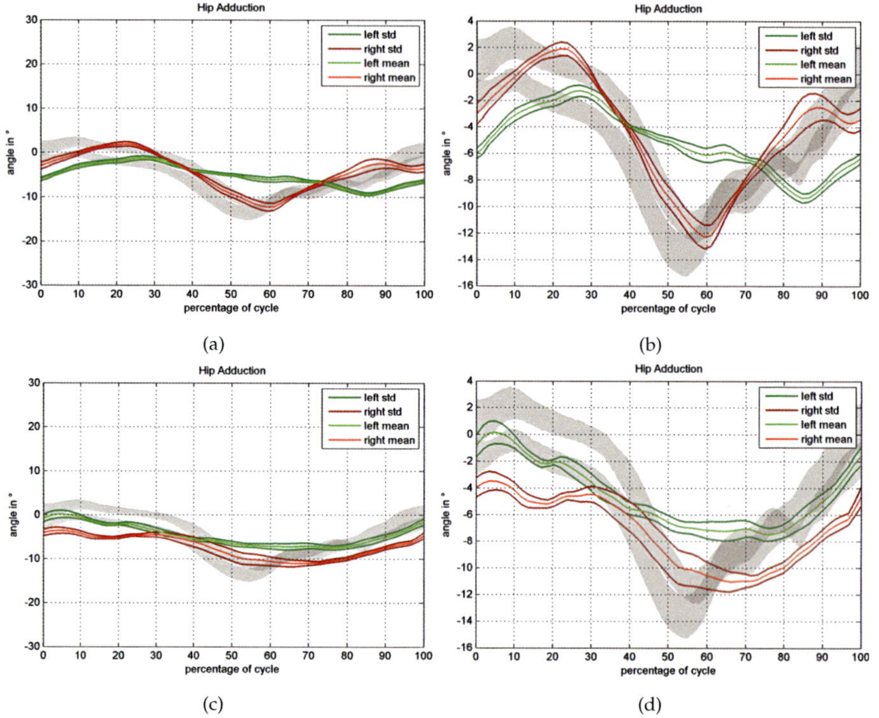

Figure 6.11: Trajectories of the hip adduction angles. The hip adduction is the angle between the thigh and the pelvis in the body's frontal plane.

Figure 6.11 shows the hip adduction. The hip adduction refers to the angle between the thigh and the pelvis in the body's frontal plane (see figure 6.5(a) and (b)). The determined hip adduction angle coarsely reflects the trend of the reference trajectories. The trajectories show a global minimum at about 50% of the gait cycle. Especially the right leg hip adduction angle trajectories reflect the reference trajectories. The minimum at the end of the stance phase at 40% to 60% of the gait cycle is less pronounced for the left hip adduction angle trajectories. The hip adduction is characterized by a absolute angle range of 18°. Although the hip adduction of the left leg deviate between 40% and 85% of the gait cycle by absolute 4°, the basic trend of the hip adduction equals to the reference trajectory. For a discussion about the causes for the deviations, the following section 6.2.3 presents an experiment which reduces the different influences on the measurement and therefore allows for a assessment of the error causes.

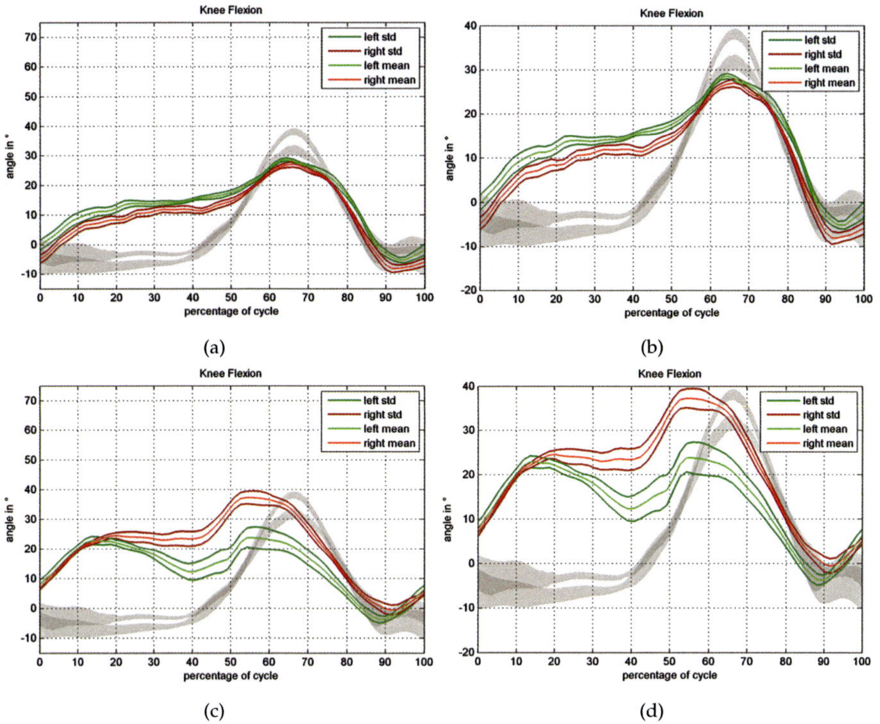

Figure 6.12: Trajectories of the knee flexion angle.

Figure 6.12 shows the knee flexion trajectories. These determined joint angle trajectories develop differently in comparison to the reference knee flexion trajectories. The determined knee flexion trajectories increase right after the initial heel contact. Such an increase of the knee flexion right at after the initial heal contact is normal for walking due to the weight acceptance. In this case the reference data does not show such a peak. This peak can be explained the fact that the clothes disturb depth data so that the depth data does not reflect the body beneath the clothes.

The determined knee flexion remains at a moderate high and passes correctly into the flexion peak at the contra lateral foot initial heel contact. The extension of the knee during swing phase equals the reference data up to the initial heel contact. For a discussion about the causes for the deviations, the following section 6.2.3 presents an experiment which reduces the different influences on the measurement and therefore allows for a assessment of the error causes.

6.2.2 Gait Symmetry

The figure 6.13 demonstrates the capability of the system to capture the symmetry of the gait. Because the symmetry shows itself in the lateral movements due to the weight takeover from one leg to the other, just the lateral position is shown. The gray area represents the reference data while the red graphs represent the joint position extracted with the realized system. For a discussion about the causes for the deviations, the following section 6.2.3 presents an experiment which reduces the different influences on the measurement and therefore allows for a assessment of the error causes.

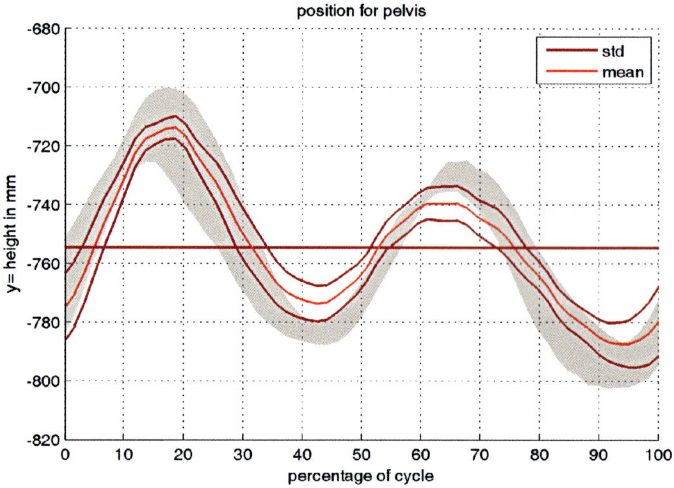

Figure 6.13: Position of the pelvis center in frontal plane giving an impression about the gait symmetry. Because the symmetry shows itself in the lateral movements due to the weight takeover from one leg to the other, just the lateral position is shown. The gray area represents the reference data while the red graphs represent the joint position extracted with the realized system.

6.2.3 Evaluation

In the previous sections the results of the developed system are presented. The determined gait parameter trajectories reflect the trend of the reference trajectories, but sometimes deviate significantly. The causes for these deviations are found on the one hand within the realized system and on the other hand within the reference data generation. The different error sources are:

1. joint angle error transfer 2. lateral sample rate 3. depth data accuracy 4. soft tissue artefacts	error sources originated in realized system
5. marker displacement 6. different model 7. marker center determination	error sources originated in reference data generation

The influences of these error sources on the determined gait parameters are investigated on the base of an experiment which reduces certain error sources and allows for their separate assessment. The scheme of the experiment setup is described together with the explanations of the different error sources. After the description of the experiment its results are discussed to identify the significant error sources of the determined gait parameters from section 6.2.1.

1st error source *'joint angle error transfer'*:
The transfer of joint angle errors origins in the kinematic coupling of the body model segments. This means that one joint's angle error is passed to another joint along the kinematic chain. A good example for this is the pelvis. If it is tilted to the front or the back, the hip flexion angle is directly affected by this. Because of the kinematic coupling of the body segments, angle errors can be aggregated over connected body segments within their degrees of freedom.
In order to minimize this error source within the experiment, just one joint angle is captured and the neighborging joints' location are kept steady. Because especially the knee angle showed a significant deviation (see figure 6.12), the experiment focuses on the knee joint. Thereby, the knee joint is captured from the front view as in the demonstrator scenario *HapticWalker* so that the same situation is present. The figure 6.14 shows some images of the experiment sequence to get an impression about the movements. The distance between the depth camera and the right leg ranges between 1.0m and 1.7m.

2nd error source *'lateral sample rate'*:
Another error source is the low lateral sample rate due to the currently relatively low 2D resolution of the TOF cameras (160 × 120 pxl for the *PMD [vision] 19k* and 320 × 240 pxl extrapolated from a smaller resolution for the *3DVSystems ZCam*). The lateral sample rate describes the lateral distribution density of the data points on the human body that are captured by the TOF camera. Because the determination of the joint angles is performed by means of a regression of the 3D body model segments and the 3D point cloud, the number of sample points per surface unit influences the regression result. Here, a greater number leads to more robust results in the context of depth data inaccuracy compensation. This means that fewer 3D points lead to an increased liability of the gait parameter determination to depth data inaccuracies. Therefore, the error caused through the low sample rate is highly related to the error that is caused by noise or systematic errors on the depth data. This is because outliers have a higher over-all weight within a low number of samples than within a high number of samples.
Because the resolution of the camera is fix, the sample rate is increased instead by capturing the object at a close distance because of the central projection of cameras. Because of the close distance, only a part of the full body is captured. This closer distance effects that e. g. the thigh is sampled by 5850 pxl instead of 765 pxl of the sequences taken for gait parameter determination from section 6.2.1. This corresponds to an increase of 764% of the number of sample points. Although at first view 765 pxl seems to be a high num-

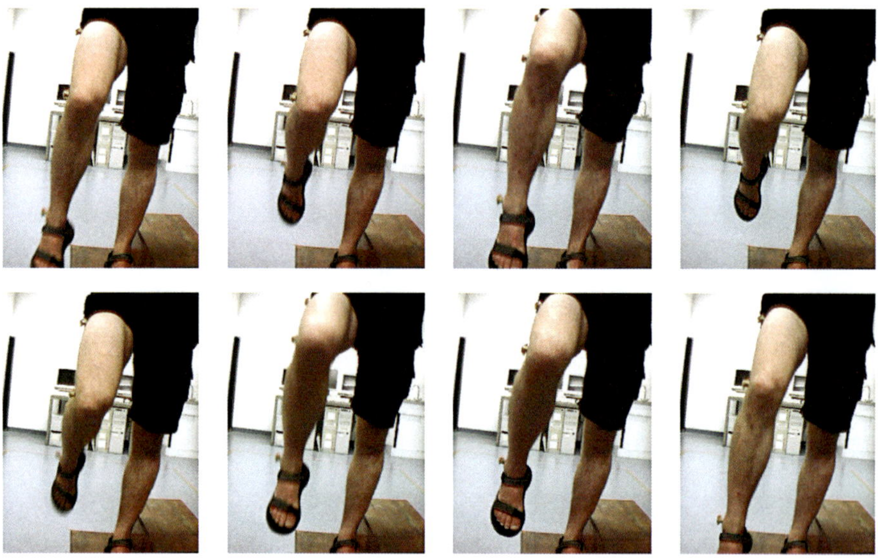

Figure 6.14: Sample images of the experiment sequence.

ber of sample points, a 764% higher sample point number is favorable for the regression. However, technical advances will increase the sample rate because upcoming versions of TOF cameras will provide a much higher resolution. At the moment resolutions of 200×200 pxl are on the market. Currently, there are appraisals about a resolution of 1 mega-pixel for TOF cameras.

3rd error source *'depth data accuracy'*:
There are different aspects of depth data accuracy. One is the noise (see section 4.1.3). The angle error caused by noise is strongly related to the lateral sample rate and depends on the amount of the noise and the visible surface of the considered body segment. This is because the body segments of the model are fitted into the 3D point cloud by means of a regression and the farther the incorporated 3D points are, the more stable is the regression result.
A reduction of the influence of the noise is achieved by also capturing the object at closer distance so that the signal-to-noise-ratio (SNR) of the depth data is increased. Due to the closer distance also the visible surface of the 3D body model increases. Therefore, the regression of the 3D body model and the 3D point cloud is supported by a greater number of data points and noise is averaged out.
Another aspect of the depth data accuracy is the inaccuracy due to variations of the object's reflectivities. Within this work methods are developed that compensate for this and reduce the average of the error from 0.20 m to less than 0.01 m (see section 4.1.4). But objects with a low reflectivity lead to a low SNR and a higher degree of noise. Therefore, an object with a uniform high reflectivity is considered.
In this context it shall be noted that technical advances will yield TOF cameras that out-of-the-box already show a reduced amount of noise.
Another aspect is the distortion of the depth data through the markers of the marker-based system. This is because of the fact that markers are omnireflective which is also the case for IR-light that is used by the TOF camera for illumination. Therefore, markers are overexposed and appear as bright dots in the depth image which corresponds to a depth that is closer than the actual one.
To compensate for this in the experiment a marker-set for the right leg is created which uses positions for the markers that are not directly visible for the TOF-camera and capable of modeling the knee flexion angle, though. This is necessary because a predefined marker-set, like the most commonly used *Plug-In-Gait*-marker-set which comes with the *Vicon*®-system, has predefined marker positions that are visible from the front view from which the TOF camera captures the patient. See section 8.1 for a visualization of the marker positions of the *Plug-In-Gait*-marker-set. The created marker-set is depicted in figure 6.15(a) with the markers illustrated as white circles.

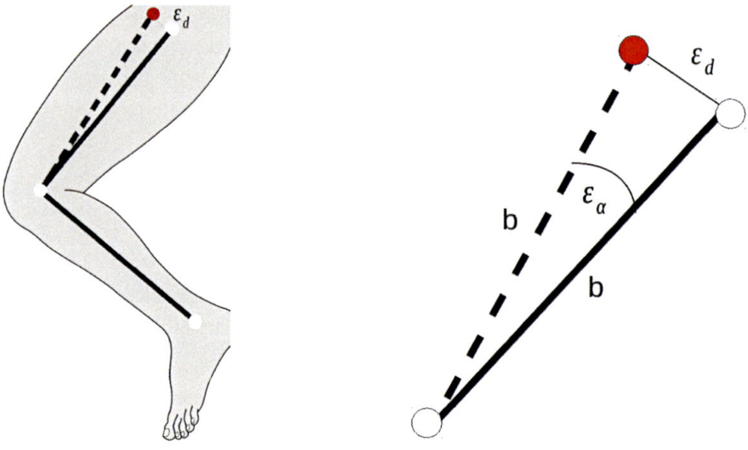

Figure 6.15: Marker-set for knee flexion angle determination for the experiment. The markers are depicted as white circles. ϵ_α represents the angle error between thigh and shank for a given bone length b. The model forms the base for the error approximation of some of the error sources. The value ϵ_d corresponds to the distance error of the different error sources, like e. g. the marker displacement. Figure (b) is a zoomed version of figure (a).

4th error source *'soft tissue artefacts'*:
The clothes also influence the joint angle measurement. This is because clothes represent soft tissues that tend to move independently in relation to the underlying body. This easily results in a deviation of the depth of a few centimeters especially at the lower trousers leg and the folds at the pelvis. The angle error due to this can be approximated. The geometric background for this error approximation is depicted in figure 6.15. If assuming the depth data error ϵ_d to be 0.05m at the pelvis, the knee angle error $\epsilon_\alpha(\epsilon_d, b)$ introduced by this can be approximated through $\epsilon_\alpha(\epsilon_d, b) = 2 \cdot \arcsin(\frac{\epsilon_d}{b})$ where b represents the length of the thigh and the shank. With a depth data error of $\epsilon_d = 0.05m$ for ankle and pelvis and a thigh and shank length of $b = 0.45m$, the angle error caused by the clothes sums up to 12.74°.
In the experiment this error source is minimized by wearing short trousers. Therefore the depth data directly samples the leg and not the clothes that cover the leg.

5th error source *'marker displacement'*:
The 'marker displacement' is an error source that relates to the reference data generation. The accuracy of the reference data depends on how accurate the markers are positioned with respect to the marker-set. This is because the joint angles are inferred from the

markers' positions. Therefore, marker displacement forms an error source.
Figure 6.15 depicts the used marker-set for approximate computation of the angle error that results from marker displacement. To simplify matters the displacement *'disp'* of the top marker that is tangential to the line towards the knee marker with a constant line distance b. The angle error ϵ_α can be approximated with $\epsilon_\alpha(\epsilon_d, b) = 2 \cdot \arcsin(\frac{\epsilon_d}{b})$ (see figure 6.15(b) for geometric background). For an exemplary worst case scenario with a displacement of $\epsilon_d = 0.02m$ and a line distance $b = 0.45m$ as an average thigh length the angle error would result to $\epsilon_\alpha = 5.09°$. This means that the angle error introduced through marker displacement is less than $5.09°$ when a maximum displacement of $d = 0.02m$ is assumed.
Because the markers are just stuck on the body, their position on the body varies due to the soft tissue artifacts. But this can be assumed to be small because of the relatively small accelerations of the considered movements.

6th error source *'different model'*:
Another error source is that the model used for reference data generation and the model of the realized system vary in the position of the joints. This is especially the case when the model is moving. The model of the realized system has fixed joint positions whereas the joint positions of the *Plug-In-Gait*-model varies the joint positions according to the model's pose. This can be interpreted similarly to the marker misplacement. Therefore, a joint position deviation of $\epsilon_{jp} = 0.015m$ results is a angle error of $\epsilon_\alpha = 3.82°$. To reduce the influence of differing models, in the experiment a model for the knee is created that corresponds to the model used by the to be evaluated system.

7th error source *'marker center determination'*:
Additionally to the possible error introduced by the marker displacement, there is the issue that the position of the markers is measured inaccurately by the *Vicon*®-system. The positioning measurement error results from digitalization and partial occlusions of the markers so that the center of the marker cannot be determined properly. This additionally affects the joint position and, therefore, the joint angle measurement for reference data generation. The maximum angle error that results from this cause is less than the marker displacement introduced error, because the positioning error is always less than the radius of the used markers. If for example the marker, whose diameter is 0.01m, is occluded so that only half of it is visible from the *Vicon*®-camera perspective, the positioning error of the marker center is less than the marker's radius. This would contribute a maximum angle error of $\epsilon_\alpha = 2.546°$ for the considered sample scenario to the overall angle error.

ERROR SOURCE	ANGLE ERROR ϵ_α [°]
joint angle error transfer	-
lateral sample rate	2.50°
depth data accuracy	2.50°
soft tissue artefacts	12.74°
marker displacement	5.09°
different model	3.82°
marker center determination	2.55°
SUM OF ANGLE ERRORS	29.20°

Table 6.6: Approximations of the knee flexion angle errors for the different error sources.

The table 6.6 lists these approximations for the different error sources. The 'joint angle error transfer' is not approximated because only one joint is considered within the experiment and therefore no transfer of an angle error can occur.

In the following the results of the experiment are presented. With these results and with the above approximations of the different error sources the causes of the deviations of the angle errors form section 6.2.1 are inferred.

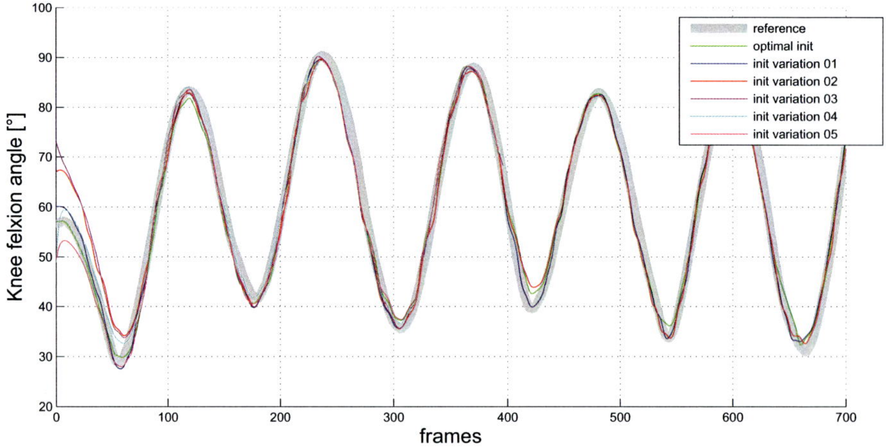

Figure 6.16: Right leg knee flexion angle of the experiment with sample images shown in figure 6.14. Each plot represents a different run on the same depth data of the realized system with a varied model initialization. The gray line is the reference data which was captured simultaneously with the markerbased *Vicon*®-system.

The figure 6.16 shows the results of the experiment. Shown is the knee flexion angle of the right leg over frames. The gray thick graph corresponds to the reference data, which was captured with the markerbased *Vicon*® system. The colored solid thin graphs correspond to the knee flexion angles that were determined with the developed system for different runs. Thereby, each run differs in the initializations of the model. The green graph represent the run which was initialized with a perfectly aligned model. The other graphs start with model initializations that do not properly represent the 3D point cloud. Thereby, the angular parameterization of the model was varied, the model segment's sizes, etc. were not modified.
The figure demonstrates that the determined knee flexion angles equal the reference data and, therefore, that the realized system is capable to accurately determine the knee joint angle. Additionally, the figure shows that the determined knee flexion angles equal the reference data regardless of the body model's knee angle initialization. This demonstrates that the system is capable to recover from bad initializations which is important especially when the realized system lost track due to occlusions and needs to recover. It can be seen that the full recovery of all bad initializations is achieved after about 70 frames.
The residua of the determined angle trajectories and the reference total to a mean of $\bar{m} = 0.34°$ with a standard deviation of $\bar{\sigma} = 0.95°$. The first 100 frames are not taken into account for this computation because these frames are needed to compensate the varied initializations of the model and do not reflect the accuracy of the determined angles. The first frames of the figure 6.16 are zoomed to demonstrate the converging of the joint angle towards the reference in figure 6.17. The figure shows that bad initializations of up to 20° are recovered with the realized system.

The results of the experiment demonstrate that the realized system is capable to accurately determine the knee flexion angle for the considered experiment setup. Because the knee flexion angle trajectory showed a significant deviation from the reference trajectory in the demonstrator scenario (see figures 6.12), the difference in the setup with respect to the different error source is the error source that causes the angle error. Therefore, the reason for the deviation between determined angle and reference angle trajectory in figures 6.12 has to be found within the error sources that were suppressed for the experiment. A comparison of the error approximation from table 6.6 and the figures 6.12 is carried out in the following to identify the causing error source.

The angle error which is measured in the demonstrator scenario has its maximum peak for the gait cycle at $\approx 30°$ (see figure 6.12). This equals to the sum of the approximations of 29.20° so that the error peak could result from the described error sources. But because 29.20° is a worst-case approximation, this would only explain the error peak from the figures 6.12. But the knee flexion angle error varies throughout the gait cycle. Therefore, the

variations of the different error sources must be considered.
The error sources *'marker displacement'* and *'marker center determination'* are nearly constant. Therefore, these error sources can only explain nearly constant errors. The same counts for the *'depth data accuracy'* and *'lateral sample rate'* for which reason the variation must result from the remaining error sources: *'joint angle error transfer'*, *'soft tissue artefacts'* and *'different model'*. *'different model'*, just by its maximum value of 3.82°, provides the smallest theoretically possible range for variation. This leads to the conclusion that the *'joint angle error transfer'* and the *'soft tissue artefacts'* are the both major responsible contributions for the angle error deviations from figure 6.12. These two error sources represent the both most important leverages for angle error reduction.
The temporal phase shift of the angle trajectory's characteristics with respect to the reference can only be explained by the *'joint angle error transfer'* (see figure 6.10). This error source can be reduced by reducing the flexibility of the model's degrees of freedom. But this would limit the potential of the system to capture pathological movements because this decreases the sensitivity of the model. But because the objective of realized system is to detect pathological gait features, the used body model has as less limitations as possible.

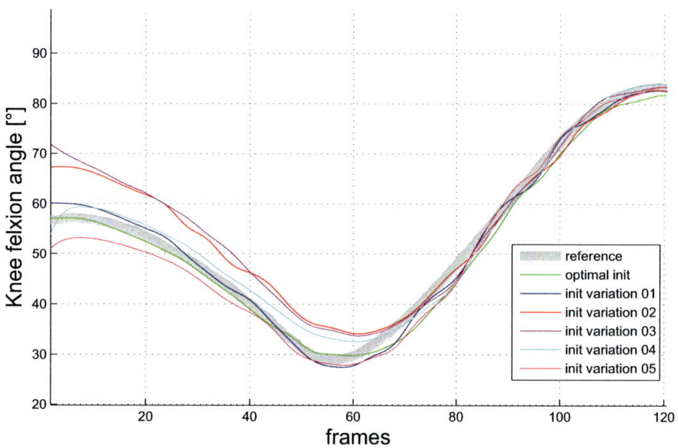

Figure 6.17: The first 120 frames of the figure 6.16 to demonstrate the potential of the realized system to recover from bad model initializations. It can be noticed that for all model initialization variations the system converges towards the reference knee flexion angle.

6.3 Clinical Applicability

The four objectives for the 3rd criterion 'Clinical Applicability' (see chapter 3) are system complexity, setup time, clinical acceptance and processing rate. The first three are handled in section 6.3.1. The processing rate is handled separately in section 6.3.2, because the 'corresponding point correction' stage was newly introduced. Section 6.3.3 gives a summarized evaluation of all required criterions.

6.3.1 System Complexity, Setup Time and Clinical Acceptance

For the applicability in clinical environment the system complexity is important. It mainly relates to the sensor system complexity, because this is the variable part of the system in terms of space requirement.
Therefore, to minimize the system complexity, just one single-view sensor is used. Due to the single view nature of TOF and standard 2D cameras, both their space requirements are equal, but the TOF camera outperforms in terms of the data, since providing depth data. This is an advantage over the widely-used multi-camera approaches that require much more space.
Additional to these arguments, there are further reasons to select the single-view TOF camera. The multi-camera system approach applying *SfS* is simply not suited for the demonstrator scenario *HapticWalker*. This is because it needs an uncovered view for all cameras to be able to generate accurate volumetric data which is hindered by the bars and the therapy suspension of the *HapticWalker* (see figure1.2).
The fact that a markerless approach is chosen has two advantages. First the gait of the patient is not influenced by any attachment of measurement technology. Second a short set-up time is achieved, because little preparations have to be done before the measurement.
The clinical acceptance of the developed system is given. The gait parameters are graphically presented over time as gait tarjectory plots, which makes interpretation easy for the clinical staff (see figure 6.6 as example).

6.3.2 Processing Rate

Another criterion for the clinical applicability is the processing rate of the system. The processing rate corresponds to the time that is needed to retrieve gait parameters of the depth images.
For the ICP-method the processing rate linearly depends on the number of iterations

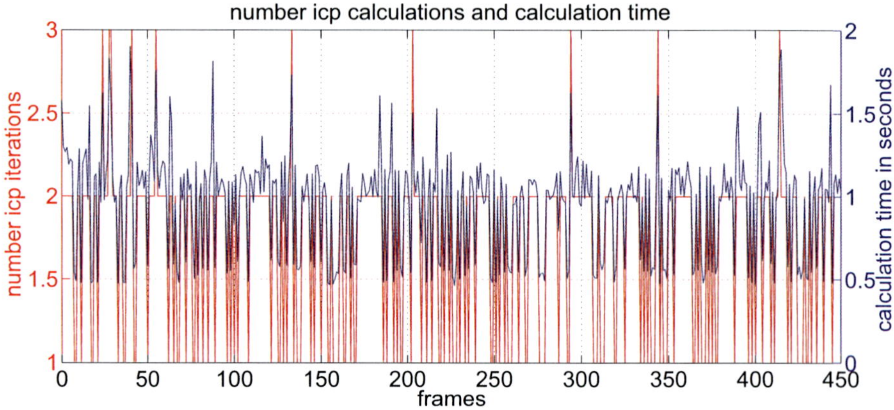

Figure 6.18: Number of ICP iterations and the corresponding processing time over frames.

which itself depend on the body movement between two subsequent frames. The bigger the movement the more iterations are needed to align the model and the 3D point cloud. Figure 6.18 shows the number of ICP iterations and the time needed for these iterations. The blue graph refers to the time and the red graph to the number of ICP-iterations. The mean number of iterations is 1.7548 with a standard deviation of 0.4529. The corresponding processing time averages to 794.6 ms for one frame with a standard deviation of 224.2ms.

In the following, the performance of the two staged corresponding point determination approach which is introduced in section 4.2.7 is presented. The main concept of the two stages is that the default corresponding point determination that determines the point correspondences on the base of the closest Euclidean distances is extended by an additional pre-stage. This corresponding point correction stage corrects the corresponding point by incorporating additionally to the closest Euclidean distance the orientation of the distance vector. The motivation for this 'corresponding point correction'-stage is to reduce the number of iterations because the corrected corresponding points lead to a faster convergence of the ICP.

To evaluate the performance of the additional stage, the ICP was run on the same data set with and without the additional 'corresponding point correction'-stage. The figure 6.19 shows the according results and demonstrates the performance. The figure 6.19(a) shows the ICP iterations and the time consumption without applying the additional 'corresponding point correction'-stage. The figure 6.19(b) shows the same, but in this case with applying the additional stage. It can be seen that the average ICP-iterations can

be reduced through additional stage. Just applying the standard corresponding point determination in the ICP results in a mean of 1.5377 of the number of ICP-iterations with a standard deviation of 1.5308. By applying the additional 'corresponding point correction'-stage a mean of 1.3358 of the number of ICP-iterations with a standard deviation of 0.9256 was achieved. This reduces the calculation time by 21.65% of the time needed if only the standard 'corresponding point determination'-stage is applied.
These results are generated on a standard PC with an Intel Core Duo with 2.33GHz and 2GB RAM- The operating system was Windows XP SP3.

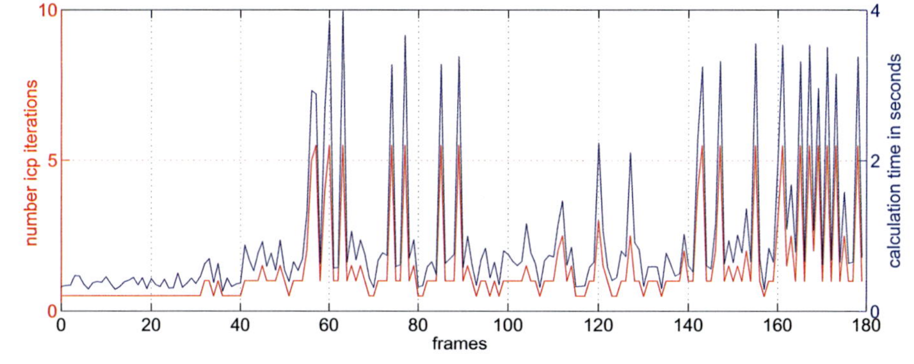

(a)

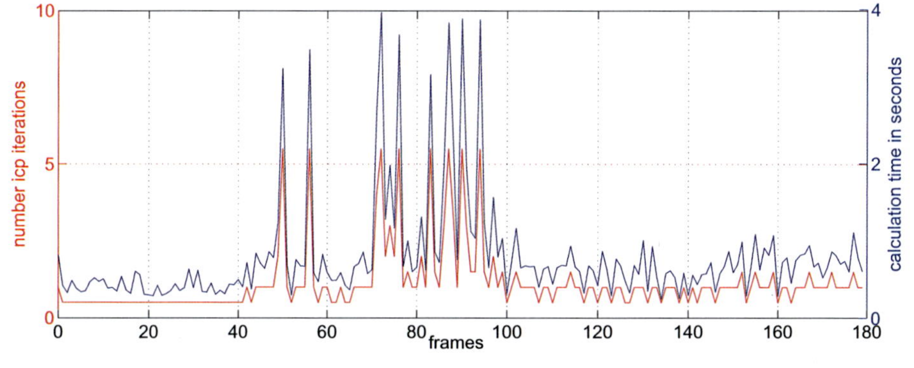

(b)

Figure 6.19: Number of ICP-iterations and corresponding calculation time, in (a) **without** applying the additional 'corresponding point correction' stage and in (b) **with** applying the additional 'corresponding point correction' stage. The figure (b) shows a reduction of the mean number of iterations.

6.3.3 Evaluation

In the following the 4 criteria of the 'Clinical Applicability' are evaluated.

1. System Complexity: As already stated, the space demand of this approach is much less compared to current multi camera approaches. In this work the TOF camera is located at a height of 2.2 m so that the camera can be attached under the ceiling which reduces space requirements even further. So the single camera approach is a very important step for the practical clinical use.

2. Setup Time: The advantages of the markerless approach are obvious. Form medical perspective, the gait of the patient is not altered which is important for an objective gait quality assessment. Additional the procedure of attaching the markers is not needed anymore and thus meeting the tight schedule of clinical personal. The markerless approach is also a very important step for the practical clinical use.

3. Clinical Acceptance: The gait parameters are graphically presented over the time as gait trajectory plots in the same style as existing commercial systems. The graphical presentation makes interpretation easy for the clinical personal, so this objective is met.

4. Processing Rate: A high processing rate is desired, so that the gait parameter trajectories are available as quick as possible. Optimal would be real-time processing, i.e., that the frame is fully processed before the next frame is captured by the TOF camera. At real-time processing, the determined gait parameters always reflect the actual joint angels of the stroke patient.
   Of course for the processing rate is depending on the performance of the target hardware and software concepts. The 'corresponding point correction'-stage was introduced to improve processing rate by reducing the number of iterations of the ICP method and thus reducing the hardware requirements. Figure 6.19 shows the number of ICP-iterations and the processing rate with and without the 'corresponding point correction'-stage. It showed that the 'corresponding point correction'-stage is capable to reduce the number of ICP-iterations in average by about 20%, which reduces post processing time. But already the current minimal processing time per frame is still about 900ms, which is still far from real-time processing demands. For real-time 30 frames need to be processed per second, resulting in a frame processing time of 33ms. So currently the gait trajectories can only be determined by post processing of the captured images. Real-time processing needs higher hardware performance.

7 Conclusion and Outlook

Because of the demographic development, the amount of stroke patients of now approx. 250 000 incidents only in Germany will further increase. This leads to an immense future burden on the health systems. Therefore the rehabilitaton therapy has to become as effective as possible to reduce costs.

An approach to achieve this is the continuous patient-adaptive gait therapy, in which the therapy progress is measured and provided to the therapists to adjust the therapy accordingly. Currently available systems have disadvantages that permit pratical clinical everyday use for stroke patients. Therefore in this work a system is presented that determines gait parameters for continous patient-adaptive gait therapy while addressing at first stage the prerequisites for an application in clinical use. The system uses a single view TOF range imaging camera because of its low complexity and the resulting small space requirement. The system works without the need to attach markers on the patient's body which reduces the set-up time enormously when automatically initialized which is not addressed within this work.

Because the depth data provided by the TOF camera out-of-the-box is not applicable for gait parameter determination, the depth data has to be corrected. The proposed methods reduce the distance error by 40% to about 10 mm, which meets the prerequisites of the considered task. The depth data enhancement comprises four stages that cover different areas. The first stage addresses the distortion of the optical path through lense distortion. In the second stage the noise of the depth data is reduced. The third 'incident light' stage reduces the dependence of the object's reflectivity on the depth measurement by exploiting knowledge about the characteristics of the TOF camera. This knowledge was experimentally gained by analysis of the raw data of the TOF cameras for different targets with known reflectivity. The correction of the reflectivity induced error incorporates an estimate of the object's reflectivity. For the *PMD [vision] 19k* the appropriate Look-up-Table is selected on the base of the estimate and for the *3DVSystems ZCam* the estimate is used as a scaling factor. The fourth stage identifies 'flying pixels' which result from the lateral undersampling of the objects at depth discontinuities and discards them. Additionally, the illumination source of the TOF camera is modeled because the self-illumination of the TOF camera results in an inhomogeneous illumination of the scene.

The system applies a deterministic model-based approach to determine the gait parameters from a sequence of corrected depth data frames. For each frame the 3D human body model is parameterized so that it corresponds to the depth data and therefore reflects the body posture of the patient. For this purpose a 3D body model is taken which features the degrees of freedom that are necessary to reflect the relevant gait parameters. The 3D body model is continuously updated for every frame with the captured data. This is performed through a regression of the 3D human body model of the previous frame into the newly captured 3D point cloud with the ICP-algorithm. As preparation for this the $2\frac{1}{2}$D data are transformed to 3D and segmented with respect to the body model segments they correspond to. The segmentation is performed partially in 2D image space and partially in 3D space. In 2D image space the segmentation is accomplish by a projection of the 3D model into the depth data and exploiting lateral distances. In 3D space the 3D Euclidean distance is used for segmentation.
Since the 3D model to 3D point cloud regression does not cover rotational movements, additionally, unique corners are identified in the 2D image space and dynamically projected onto the model in 3D. These corners are tracked in 3D over subsequent frames to cover rotation. The gait parameters are then determined from the relative poses between the body segments. An additional rise of the robustness of the synthesis is increased by the tracking of body parts in case of sparse data. For the hands this is achieved with a non-parametric skin-color initialized tracker that incorporates the depth data.

The realized system was evaluated with the demonstrator scenario *HapticWalker*. For the evaluation the determined gait parameters were compared with reference gait parameters that were captured with a markerbased *Vicon*®-system. It showed that the realized system is capable to determine the relevant gait parameters. The comparison demonstrated that the determined gait parameter trajectories reflect the trend of the reference trajectories. But sometimes the determined gait parameters deviate significantly from the reference. The causes for these deviations are found on the one hand within the realized system and on the other hand within the reference data generation.
The error sources originated in the realized system can be traced back to two relevant error sources. By far the biggest error source is the effect of cloth on the distance measure of the TOF camera. Another error source is given by the modeling because it occurs that joint angle errors transfer from one angle to neighboring body segments which is related to the relatively low pixel resolution of the TOF cameras. Therefore, future generations of the TOF cameras will contribute to this through a higher resolution and data quality.

An experiment was carried out which reduces the error sources in order to demonstrate the functionality of the realized system. The determined angle trajectories of the experiment demonstrate the functionality by reflecting very well the reference angle trajectories with a mean angle error of 0.34° and a standard deviation of 0.95°. The experiment demonstrates that the realized system is working when the error sources are overcome.

Because of the multifold advantages of the markerless single-view TOF camera based approach, it is important to overcome the error sources. The future work is to compensate for the clothes and has to lead towards a model that reduces the transfer of joint angle errors through the kinematic coupling of the body model segments and at the same time being capable to represent pathological patterns. Additionally, an automatic initialization needs to be integrated to profit of the markerless approach and its potential to reduce set-up time.

8 Appendix

8.1 Plug-In-Gait Marker Set

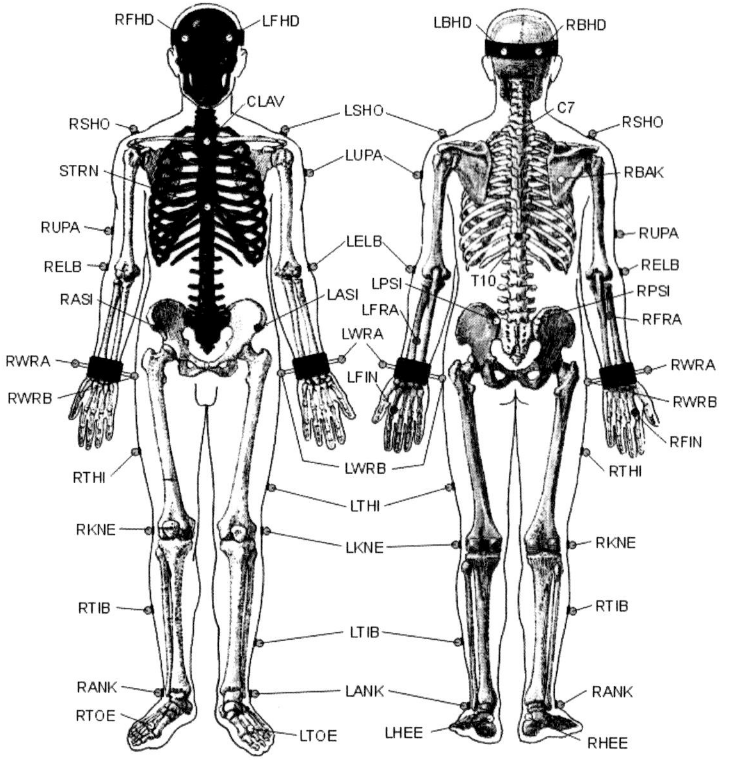

Figure 8.1: This figure shows the used marker set *'Plug-In-Gait'* taken from [100].

Bibliography

[1] Ankur Agarwal and Bill Triggs. Recovering 3d human pose from monocular images. *IEEE Trans. Pattern Anal. Mach. Intell.*, 28(1):44–58, 2006.

[2] Dragomir Anguelov, Praveen Srinivasan, Daphne Koller, Sebastian Thrun, Jim Rodgers, and James Davis. Scape: shape completion and animation of people. *ACM Trans. Graph.*, 24(3):408–416, 2005.

[3] Richard Baker. Gait analysis methods in rehabilitation. *Journal of NeuroEngineering and Rehabilitation*, 3(1):4+, March 2006.

[4] Alexandru O. Balan, Leonid Sigal, Michael J. Black, James E. Davis, and Horst W. Haussecker. Detailed human shape and pose from images. In *CVPR*. IEEE Computer Society, 2007.

[5] Herbert Bay, Tinne Tuytelaars, Van Gool, and L. Surf: Speeded up robust features. In *9th European Conference on Computer Vision*, Graz Austria, May 2006.

[6] Paul J. Besl and Neil D. McKay. A method for registration of 3-d shapes. *IEEE Trans. Pattern Anal. Mach. Intell.*, 14(2):239–256, 1992.

[7] M. Black and Y. Yacoob. Tracking and recognizing rigid and non-rigid facial motion using local parametric models of image motion. In *Proceedings of the ICCV*, pages 12–17. IEEE Computer Society, 1995.

[8] Amit Bleiweiss and Michael Werman. Fusing time-of-flight depth and color for real-time segmentation and tracking. In *Dyn3D '09: Proceedings of the DAGM 2009 Workshop on Dynamic 3D Imaging*, pages 58–69, Berlin, Heidelberg, 2009. Springer-Verlag.

[9] W. Boehler, M. Bordas Vicent, and A. Marbs. Investigating laser scanner accuracy. *XIX. th. Cipa Symposium at Antalya, Turkey, 2003*, 2003.

[10] Gunilla Borgefors. Distance transformations in digital images. *Comput. Vision Graph. Image Process.*, 34(3):344–371, 1986.

[11] J. Y. Bouguet. Camera calibration toolbox for matlab, 2008.

[12] Gary Bradski and Adrian Kaehler. *Learning OpenCV*. O'Reilly Media Inc., 2008.

[13] Gary R. Bradski. Computer vision face tracking for use in a perceptual user interface. *Intel Technology Journal*, (Q2), 1998.

[14] RA. Brand and RD. Crowninshield. Comment on criteria for patient evaluation tools. *Journal of Biomechanics*, 14(9):655., 1981.

[15] Richard A. Brand. Can biomechanics contribute to clinical orthopaedic assessments? *Iowa Orthopaedic Journal*, 9:61–64, 1989.

[16] S. Brunnstrom. *Movement Therapy in Hemiplegia*. Harper and Row, London, 1970.

[17] Roman Calow. *Markerlose Ganganalyse mit einem Multikamerasystem*. PhD thesis, Otto-von-Guericke-Universität Magdeburg, 2005.

[18] Y. Chen and G.G. Medioni. Object modeling by registration of multiple range images. 10(3):145–155, April 1992.

[19] German K. M. Cheung, Simon Baker, Cheung Simon, and Takeo Kanade. Shape-from-silhouette of articulated objects and its use for human body kinematics estimation and motion capture. 2003.

[20] J. Clark and S. Robson. Accuracy of measurements made with cyrax 2500 laser scanner against surfaces of known colour. *Geo-Imagery Bridging Continents (ISPRS 2004)*, 2004.

[21] Dorin Comaniciu, Visvanathan Ramesh, and Peter Meer. Kernel-based object tracking. *IEEE Trans. Pattern Anal. Mach. Intell.*, 25(5):564–575, 2003.

[22] Meer P. Comaniciu, D. Mean shift: A robust approach toward feature space analysis. *IEEE Trans. Pattern Analysis Machine Intell.*, 24(5):603–619, 2002.

[23] Patricia M. Davies. *Hemiplegie*, volume 2. Auflage. Springer- Verlag, 2002.

[24] R.B. Davis, S. Ounpuu, Tyburski D., and Gage J.R. A gait analysis collection and reduction technique. *Human Movement Science*, 10:575–587, 1991.

[25] Daniel F. Dementhon and Larry S. Davis. Model-based object pose in 25 lines of code. *Int. J. Comput. Vision*, 15(1-2):123–141, 1995.

[26] D. Demirdjian, T. Ko, and T. Darrell. Constraining human body tracking. In *ICCV '03: Proceedings of the Ninth IEEE International Conference on Computer Vision*, page 1071, Washington, DC, USA, 2003. IEEE Computer Society.

[27] David Demirdjian and Trevor Darrell. 3-d articulated pose tracking for untethered diectic reference. In *ICMI '02: Proceedings of the 4th IEEE International Conference on Multimodal Interfaces*, page 267, Washington, DC, USA, 2002. IEEE Computer Society.

[28] Alessandro Verri Emanuele Trucco. *Introductory Techniques for 3-D Computer Vision*. Prentice Hall.

[29] Olivier Faugeras. *Three-dimensional computer vision*. MIT Press, 1993.

[30] K. Fukunaga and L.D. Hostetler. The estimation of the gradient of a density function, with applications in pattern recognition. *IEEE Transactions on In Information Theory*, 21(1):32–40, January 1975.

[31] Liu L. Murphy M. Fuller, J. and R. Mann. A comparison of lower extremity skeletal kinematics measured using skin- and pin-mounted markers. *Human Movement Science*, 16:219–42, 1997.

[32] M. Goffredo, R.D. Seely, J.N. Carter, and M.S. Nixon. Markerless view independent gait analysis with self-camera calibration. pages 1–6, 2008.

[33] A.A. Grattarola. Volumetric reconstruction from object silhouettes: A regularization procedure. *Signal Processing*, 27(1):27–35, 1992.

[34] S.Á. Guðmundsson, H. Aanæs, and R. Larsen. Environmental effects on measurement uncertainties of time-of-flight cameras. In *International Symposium on Signals Circuits and Systems - (ISSCS 2007)*, July 2007.

[35] Ronen Gvili, Amir Kaplan, Eyal Ofek, and Giora Yahav. Depth keying. volume 5006, pages 564–574. SPIE, 2003.

[36] R. I. Hartley and A. Zisserman. *Multiple View Geometry in Computer Vision*. Cambridge University Press, ISBN: 0521540518, second edition, 2004.

[37] Herbert Hatze. *Methoden biomechanischer Bewegungsanalyse*. Österreichischer Bundesverlag, 1986.

[38] Paul S. Heckbert. A seed fill algorithm. pages 275–277, 1990.

[39] Prof. Dr. Michael Hennerici and Dr. Hansjörg Bäzner. *Gangstörungen- Grundlagen und computergestützte Ganganalyse*. Springer Verlag, 2001.

[40] Arnim Henze. *Dreidimensionale biomechanische Modellierung und die Entwicklung eines Reglers zur Simulation zweibeinigen Gehens*. PhD thesis, Fakultät für Physik der Eberhard-Karls-Universität zu Tübingen, 2002.

[41] Stefan Hesse. *Lokomotionstherapie - Ein praxisorientierter Überblick*. Hippocampus Verlag, 2007.

[42] Michael Isard and Andrew Blake. Condensation - conditional density propagation for visual tracking. *International Journal of Computer Vision*, 29(1):5–28, 1998.

[43] Rasmus R. Jensen, Rasmus R. Paulsen, and Rasmus Larsen. Analysis of gait using

a treadmill and a time-of-flight camera. In *Dyn3D '09: Proceedings of the DAGM 2009 Workshop on Dynamic 3D Imaging*, pages 154–166, Berlin, Heidelberg, 2009. Springer-Verlag.

[44] Casey K. Kerrigan Joel A. DeLisa. *Gait Analysis In The Science Of Rehabilitation*. 1998.

[45] S. X. Ju, M. J. Black, and Y. Yacoob. Cardboard people: A parameterized model of articulated motion. In *International Conference on Automatic Face and Gesture Recognition*, pages 38–44, Killington, Vermont, 1996.

[46] T. Kahlmann, F. Remondino, and H. Ingensand. Calibration for increased accuracy of the range imaging camera swissranger. In *International Archives of Photogrammetry, Remote Sensing and Spatial Information Sciences, ISPRS Commission V Symposium*, volume XXXVI, pages 136–141, 2006.

[47] Behzad Kamgar-Parsi and Behrooz Kamgar-Parsi. Matching sets of 3d line segments with application to polygonal arc matching. *IEEE Trans. Pattern Anal. Mach. Intell.*, 19(10):1090–1099, 1997.

[48] Ken-ichi Kanatani and Tsai-Chia Chou. Shape from texture: general principle. *Artif. Intell.*, 38(1):1–48, 1989.

[49] Steffen Knoop. *Interaktive Erstellung und Ausführung von Wissen für einen Servicerroboter*. PhD thesis, Universität Karlsruhe, Fakultät Informatik, November 2007.

[50] PL Kolominsky-Rabas, C. Sarti, PU. Heuschmann, C. Graf, S. Siemonsen, B. Neundoerfer, A. Katalinic, KG. Gassmann, E. Lang, and TH. Ritter von Stockert. A prospective community-based study of stroke in germany: The erlangen stroke project (espro). incidence and case fatality at 1, 3 and 12 months. *Stroke*, 29:2501–2506, 1998.

[51] Jörg Krüger, T K Lien, and Alexander Verl. Cooperation of human and machines in assembly lines. *CIRP Annals - Manufacturing Technology*, 59, 2009.

[52] Jörg Krüger and Jochen Radmer. Markerbasiertes bewegungserfassungssystem zur verbesserung der forschungsinfrastruktur zur vorbereitung und durchführung neuer forschungsvorhaben. TU-Berlin-internal funding proposal, Oktober 2008.

[53] Nickolay B. Heyer P. Krüger, J. and G. Seliger. Image based 3d surveillance for flexible man-robot-cooperation. *CIRP Annals - Manufacturing Technology*, pages 19–22, 2005.

[54] K.-D. Kuhnert and M. Stommel. Fusion of stereo-camera and pmd-camera data for real-time suited precise 3d environment reconstruction. In *Proceedings of the International Conference on Intelligent Robots and Systems*, pages 4780 – 4785, 2006.

[55] R. Lange. *3D Time-of-Flight Distance Measurement with Custom Solid-State Image Sensors in CMOS/CCD-Technology*. PhD thesis, University Siegen, 2000.

[56] A. Leardinia, L. Chiari, U. Della Croce, and A. Cappozzo. Human movement analysis using stereophotogrammetry: Part 3. soft tissue artifact assessment and compensation. *Comput. Methods Prog. Biomed.*, 21(2):212–225, February 2005.

[57] M. Lindner and A. Kolb. Lateral and depth calibration of pmd-distance sensors. In *ISVC (2)- Advances in Visual Computing, Second International Symposium*, volume 4292 of *Lecture Notes in Computer Science*, pages 524–533. Springer Verlag, 2006.

[58] M. Lindner and A. Kolb. Calibration of the intensity-related distance error of the pmd tof-camera. In *SPIE: Intelligent Robots and Computer Vision XXV*, volume 6764, pages 6764–35, September 2007.

[59] D.D. Litchi. The effects of reflecting surface material properties on time-of-flight laser scanner measurements. *Dynamic 3D Imaging (Workshop in Conjunction with DAGM 2007)*, 2007.

[60] Alberto Leardinic-Aurelio Cappozzo Lorenzo Chiaria, Ugo Della Croceb. Human movement analysis using stereophotogrammetry: Part 2: Instrumental errors. *Gait & Posture*, 21(2):197–211, Februrary 2005.

[61] David G. Lowe. Distinctive image features from scale-invariant keypoints. *International Journal of Computer Vision*, 60(2):91–110, 2004.

[62] Xuming Luan. *Experimental Investigation of Photonic Mixer Device and Development of TOF 3D Ranging Systems Based on PMD Technology*. PhD thesis, Department of Electrical Engineering and Computer Science at University of Siegen, 2001.

[63] W. N. Martin and J. K. Aggarwal. Volumetric description of objects from multiple views. In *IEEE Transactions on Pattern Analysis and Machine Intelligence*, volume PAMI-5, pages 150–158, 1983.

[64] Karl-Heinz Mauritz. *Rehabilitation nach Schlaganfall*. Kohlhammer, 1994.

[65] Stefan May, Björn Werner, Hartmut Surmann, and Kai Pervölz. 3d time-of-flight cameras for mobile robotics. In *Proceedings of the International Conference on Intelligent Robots and Systems (IROS)*, pages 790–795, Beijing, China, October 2006. IEEE Computer Society.

[66] K. McLaren. The development of the cie 1976 (l*a*b*) uniform colour space and colour-difference formula. *Journal of the Society of Dyers and Colourists*, 92, 1976.

[67] Tobias Möller, Holger Kraft, Jochen Frey, Martin Albrecht, and Robert Lange. Robust 3d measurements with pmd sensors. *Proceedings of the 1st Range Imaging Re-*

search Day at ETH Zurich, 2005.

[68] L. Mündermann, S. Corazza, and T Andriacchi. The evolution of methods for the capture of human movement leading to markerless motion capture for biomechanical applications. *Journal of NeuroEngineering and Rehabilitation*, 3(1):1–11, 2006.

[69] L. Mündermann, S. Corazza, and T.P. Andriacchi. Accurately measuring human movement using articulated icp with soft-joint constraints and a repository of articulated models. pages 1–6, 2007.

[70] L. Mündermann, S. Corazza, A. M. Chaudhari, Andriacchi T. P., Sundaresan A., and Chellappa R. Measuring human movement for biomechanical applications using markerless motion capture. *Three-Dimensional Image Capture and Applications VII. Proceedings of the SPIE*, 6056:246–255, 2006.

[71] Kirsten Götz Neumann. *Gehen verstehen, Ganganalyse in der Physiotherapie*. Georg Thieme Verlag Stuttgart - New York, 2006.

[72] Yoon-Hyuk Kim Tae-Seong Kim Nguyen Duc Thang, Young-Koo Lee. Markerless 3-d human motion capturing using a stereo camera. In Ph.D. Ed Quigley, editor, *Proceedings of the 2nd Joint ESMAC-GCMAS Conference*, Miami, Florida USA, May 12-15 2010. Gait and Clinical Movement Analysis Society (GCMAS) and European Society of Movement Analysis in Adults and Children (ESMAC), Gait and Clinical Movement Analysis Society (GCMAS) and European Society of Movement Analysis in Adults and Children (ESMAC).

[73] Wolfgang Niem. Error analysis for silhouette-based 3d shape estimation from multiple views. volume 0, 1997.

[74] N.N. Deutsches institut für normung, din 33402 - körpermaße des menschen. Technical Report 33402, Köln, 1986.

[75] J. Perry. *Gait Analysis*. Slack, 1992.

[76] Jacquelin Perry. *Ganganalyse - Norm und Pathologie des Gehens*, volume 1. Auflage. Urban und Fischer, 2003.

[77] Valerij Peters and Otmar Loffeld. A bistatic simulation approach for a high resolution 3d pmd-camera. *Dynamic 3D Vision (Workshop in Conjunction with DAGM 2007)*, 2007.

[78] PMDTechnologies-GmbH. Minisdk programming manual for 3d time of flight cameras, www.pmdtec.com. Technical report, 2005.

[79] J. Radmer, P.M. Fuste, H. Schmidt, and J. Krüger. Incident light related distance error study and calibration of the pmd-range imaging camera. In *Proceedings of IEEE*

Computer Society Conference on Computer Vision and Pattern Recognition Workshops, 2008. CVPRW '08. TOF-CV08, pages 1–6, Anchorage, Alaska, USA, July 2008. IEEE Computer Society, IEEE Computer Society.

[80] J. Radmer and J. Krüger. Moving object detection using dynamic 2 1/2d data for robot surrounding field monitoring. In J.J. Villanueva, editor, *Proceeding of the 7th Int. Conference on Visualization, Imaging, and Image Processing (VIIP 2007)*, pages 64–69, Palma de Mallorca, Spain, August 2007. IASTED, Acta Press.

[81] Jochen Radmer, Sami Hussein, and Jörg Krüger. Depth data based human motion capture for assessment of robot assisted gait rehabilitation. In *Proceedings of the First AMA-IEEE Conference on Medical Technology*. American Medical Association (AMA) and the IEEE Engineering in Medicine and Biology (EMB) Society, March 2010.

[82] Jochen Radmer, Sami Hussein, and Jörg Krüger. Marker less motion tracking for assessment of robot assisted gait rehabilitation. In Ph.D. Ed Quigley, editor, *Proceedings of the 2nd Joint ESMAC-GCMAS Conference*, Miami, Florida USA, May 12-15 2010. Gait and Clinical Movement Analysis Society (GCMAS) and European Society of Movement Analysis in Adults and Children (ESMAC), Gait and Clinical Movement Analysis Society (GCMAS) and European Society of Movement Analysis in Adults and Children (ESMAC).

[83] Jochen Radmer and Jörg Krüger. Depth data based capture of human movement for biomechanical application in clinical rehabilitation. In *Proceedings of the 5th International IEEE Computer Society Symposium on Health Informatics and Bioinformatics (HIBIT 2010)*, Lara, Antalya, Turkey, April 20-22 2010. IEEE, IEEE Computer Society.

[84] Jochen Radmer and Jörg Krüger. Ganganalyse für die klinische anwendung auf basis von tiefendaten. In T.M. Deserno, H. Handels, H.-P. Meinzer, and T. Tolxdorff, editors, *Proceedings of Bildverarbeitung für die Medizin 2010, Algorithmen – Systeme – Anwendungen*, Informatik aktuell, pages 385–390, Aachen, Germany, 14.-16. March 2010. IEEE, Gesellschaft für Informatik, Springer.

[85] Jochen Radmer, Alexander Sabov, and Jörg Krüger. Data evaluation for depth calibration of a customary pmd range imaging sensor considering objects with different albedo. In *Proceedings of the 3th. International Conference on Computer Vision Theory and Applications (VISAPP 2008)*, pages 169–173, Funchal, Portugal, January 2008. INSTICC, INSTICC PRESS.

[86] H Rapp, M Frank, FA Hamprecht, and B Jähne. A theoretical and experimental investigation of the systematic errors and statistical uncertainties of time-of-flight cameras. *Dynamic 3D Imaging (Workshop in Conjunction with DAGM 2007)*, 2007.

[87] Holger Rapp. Experimental and theoretical investigation of correlating tof-camera systems. Master's thesis, Interdisciplinary Center for Scientific Computing (IWR) - Ruprecht-Karls-University of Heidelberg, 2007.

[88] Pam Thomason Richard Baker, Jenny McGinley. *Impairment focused Interpretation: A Clinical Reasoning Approach to the interpretation and understanding of gait analysis data.*, 2010.

[89] Jessica Rose and James G. Gamble. *Human Walking*. Williams & Wilkins, 1993.

[90] E. Roux, S Bouillandb, A.-P Godillon-Maquinghena, and D Bouttens. Evaluation of the global optimisation method within the upper limb kinematics analysis. *Journal of Biomechanics*, 35(9):1279–1283, 2002.

[91] Joaquim Salvi, Carles Matabosch, David Fofi, and Josep Forest. A review of recent range image registration methods with accuracy evaluation. *Image Vision Comput.*, 25:578–596, 2007.

[92] Henning Schmidt, Cordula Werner, Stefan Hesse, Rolf Bernhardt, and Joerg Krueger. Gait rehabilitation machines based on programmable footplates. *Journal of NeuroEngineering and Rehabilitation*, 4:2+, February 2007.

[93] S. Schuon, C. Theobalt, J. Davis, and S. Thrun. High-quality scanning using time-of-flight depth superresolution. pages 1–7, 2008.

[94] D. W. Scott. *Multivariate Density Estimation*. Wiley, 1992.

[95] Jean Serra and Luc Vincent. An overview of morphological filtering. *Circuits Syst. Signal Process.*, 11(1):47–108, 1992.

[96] Jianbo Shi and Carlo Tomasi. Good features to track. In *1994 IEEE Conference on Computer Vision and Pattern Recognition (CVPR'94)*, pages 593 – 600, 1994.

[97] P. Soille. *Morphologische Bildverarbeitung*. Springer-Verlag, Berlin, Heidelberg, 1998.

[98] H. Stolze, P. Vieregge, and G. Deuschl. Gangstörungen in der neurologie. *Der Nervenarzt*, 79:485–499, 2008.

[99] 3DV Systems. Zcam operating manual. Technical report, 2008.

[100] Vicon. Plug-in-gait marker placement documentation, 2007.

[101] Vicon. Techical datasheet, 2009.

[102] S. Wachter and H.-H. Nagel. Tracking persons in monocular image sequences. *International Journal on Computer Vision and Image Understanding*, 74(3):174–192, 1999.

[103] R.L. Waters, J. Frazier, and Garland D.E. Electromyographic gait analysis before

and after operative treatment for hemiplegic equinus and equinovarus deformity. In *Journal Bone Joint Surg Am*, volume 64, pages 284–8., 1982.

[104] W. Michael Whittle. *Gait Analysis: An Introduction*. Butterworth-Heinemann, 2007.

[105] D. A. Winter. *Biomechanics and Motor Control of Human Movement*. Wiley-Interscience, New York, 2nd edition, 1990.

[106] M. Yamamoto and K. Yagishita. Scene constraintsaided tracking of human body. In *Proceedings of the Conference on Computer Vision and Pattern Recognition (CVPR'00)*, pages 151–156, Hilton Head Island, SC,, June 2000. IEEE Computer Society.

[107] Ruo Zhang, Ping-Sing Tsai, James Edwin Cryer, and Mubarak Shah. Shape from shading: A survey. *IEEE Transactions on Pattern Analysis and Machine Intelligence*, 21(8):690–706, 1999.